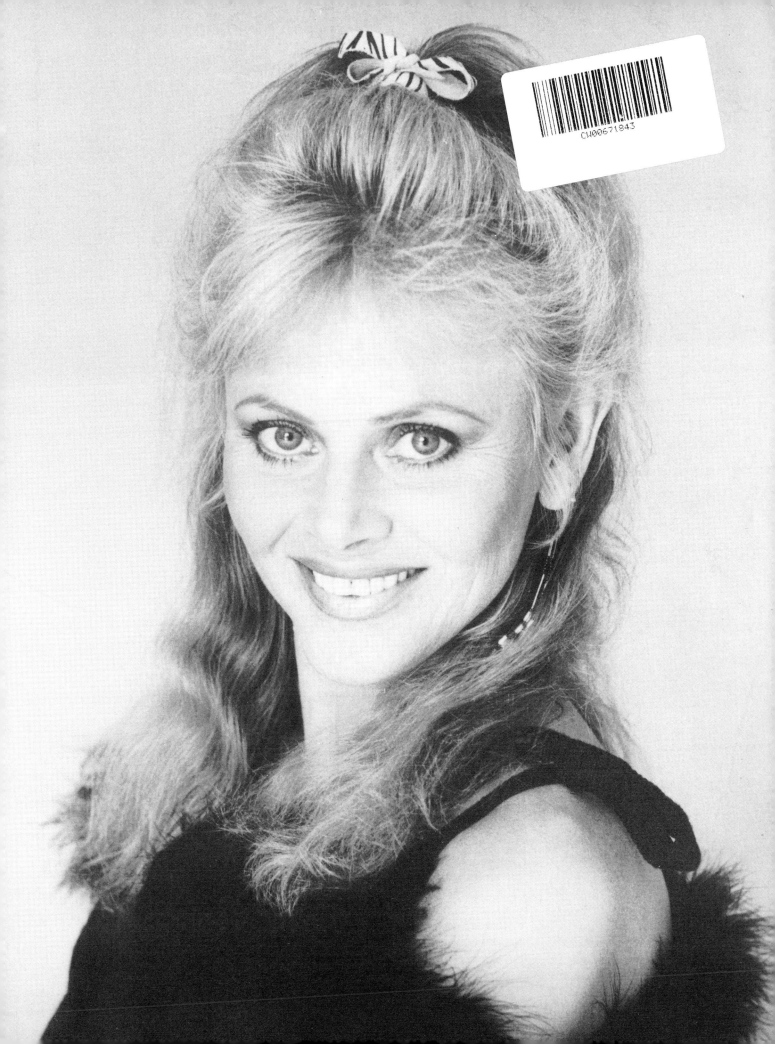

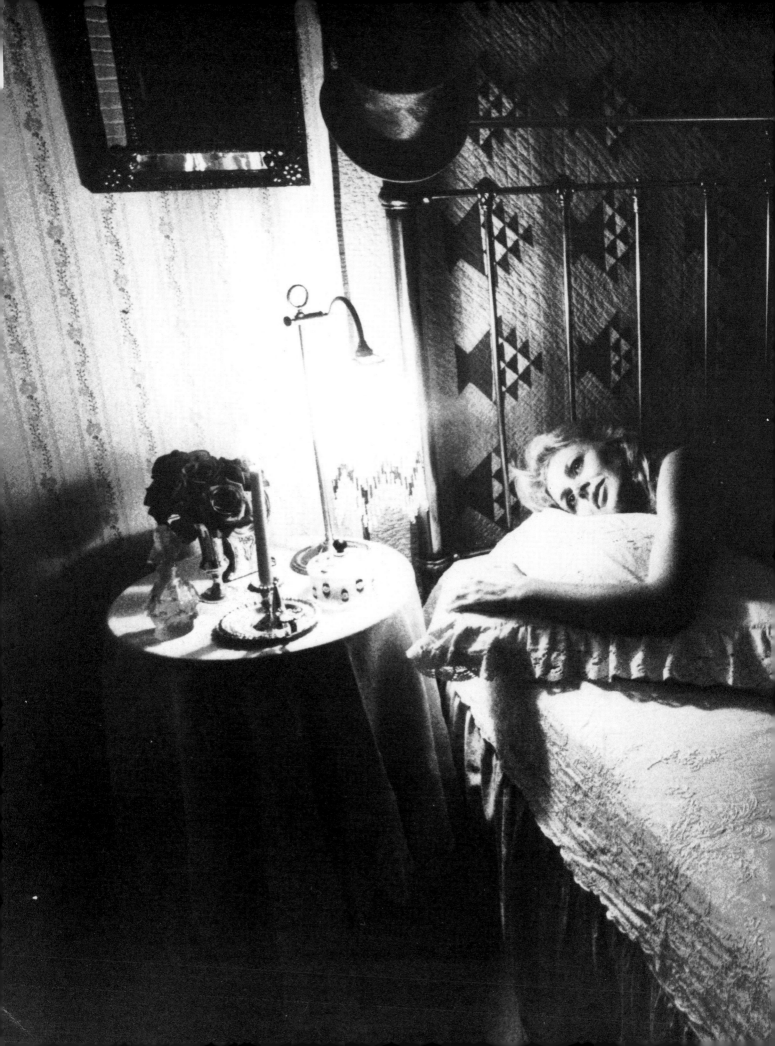

Sensual Beauty

AND HOW TO ACHIEVE IT

BRITT EKLAND

WITH

SUE RUSSELL

PHOTOGRAPHS BY

DAVID STEEN

SIDGWICK & JACKSON

LONDON

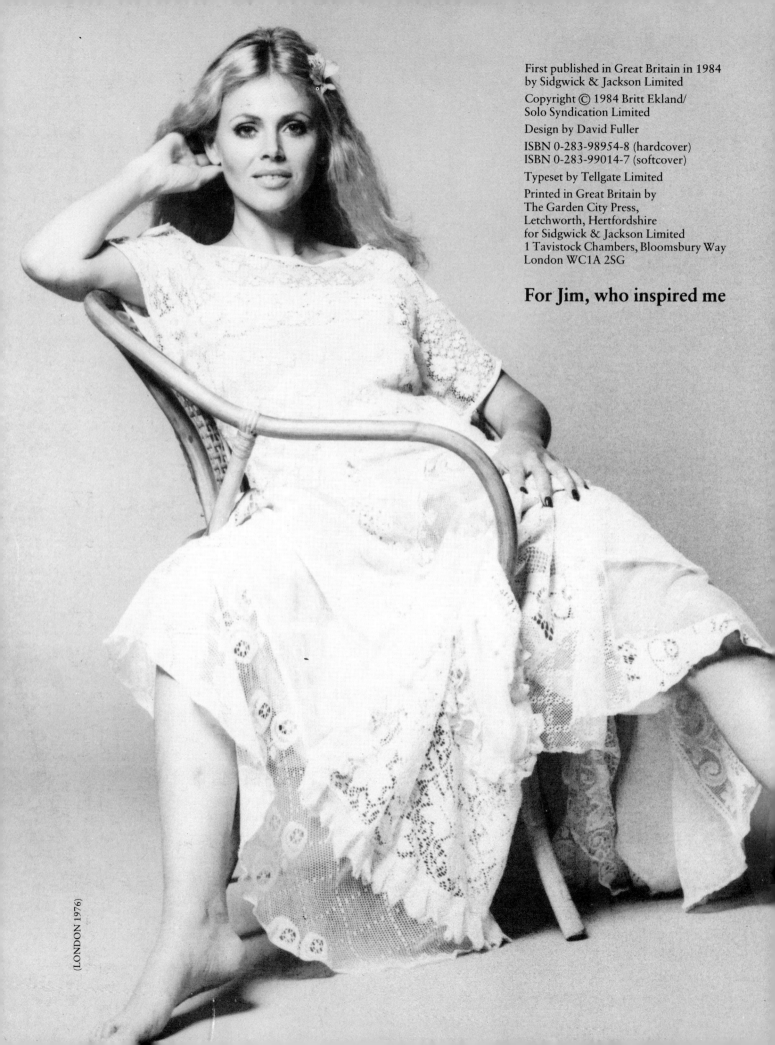

First published in Great Britain in 1984
by Sidgwick & Jackson Limited

Copyright © 1984 Britt Ekland/
Solo Syndication Limited

Design by David Fuller

ISBN 0-283-98954-8 (hardcover)
ISBN 0-283-99014-7 (softcover)

Typeset by Tellgate Limited

Printed in Great Britain by
The Garden City Press,
Letchworth, Hertfordshire
for Sidgwick & Jackson Limited
1 Tavistock Chambers, Bloomsbury Way
London WC1A 2SG

For Jim, who inspired me

(LONDON 1976)

PHOTO ACKNOWLEDGEMENTS
The very early photographs of Britt (pages 8-9 and 10-11) come from her own album. The author and publishers are grateful to Scope Features for allowing us to reproduce the twelve photographs on pages 4-5, 12-13, 15, 28-9, 73, 82, 99, 116, 117, 122-3, 128 and 135. These were taken by David Steen between 1974 and 1981. All the other photographs in the book were taken specially for it during 1983 by David Steen, and are his copyright.

AUTHOR'S ACKNOWLEDGEMENTS
This book is very much a joint effort, so I want to thank my writer Sue Russell and my photographer David Steen for managing to win my trust and capture my true image.

David and I go back to the James Bond movie, *The Man With The Golden Gun*, and I will never forget the ease and comfort I felt in the presence of this very proper-looking Englishman. He made the camera speak the truth. We have maintained a great friendship during a consistent working relationship and I feel very fortunate that he was available to bring his high standards and artistic integrity to this exciting project. Thank you, David.

Sue, who is also English, and has a long list of credits to her name, has interviewed me for several publications over the past seven years and her writing is always fair and truthful. My thoughts on how this book should be executed are perfectly represented by Sue's tremendous journalistic experience and her own beauty knowledge. She also possesses the amazing ability to retain my informal expressions and to write the way I speak. Thank you, Sue.

Britt Ekland
Los Angeles
November 1983

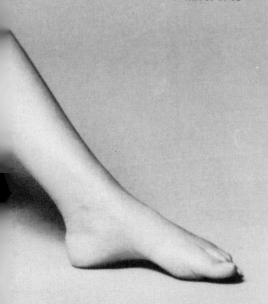

CONTENTS

FOREWORD /
FROM ME TO YOU

I don't deny that I have led a tremendously eventful life. I have done a lot of things that most people only dream about. But contrary to popular belief, I do not lead a round-the-clock jet-set existence, perpetually rubbing shoulders with other celebrities. Nor do I languish in the lap of luxury. Sometimes I do, but far from always.

Yes, I have been lucky, but I have also been broke and just about as low as a human being can get. Being famous hasn't meant I have been spared anything. I have gone from overweight to anorexia to bingeing and finally to healthy eating. I have been pregnant, given birth, been a mother alone, brought up a child alone, survived broken love affairs and been through a hell of a lot on every physical, emotional and intellectual level.

I am naturally curious about everything connected with the body, with the ageing process and with disease – in part because I was married to Peter Sellers who, it is now known, suffered eight massive heart attacks, but also because my mother had cancer. Her weight dropped from 105lb to 50lb and she was given five weeks to live, but she survived. These experiences affected me deeply.

I have achieved things with my own body that at one time I would not have thought possible. I have proved to myself that I can lose weight and more important, keep it off. I have passed the big 'forty' and so far required no plastic surgery. My body is still looking young and taut and so is my skin, partly due to my Swedish genes, no doubt. Through exercising and a healthy diet I have the energy level, I swear, of someone fifteen years younger. I feel good about myself and proud of the way I look, and that, I believe, is the real key to being a sensual woman.

I get plenty of compliments. My man is always amazed at how soft my skin is, for instance. I do take good care of it and I credit my daily shower routine with keeping it like a baby's. Men admire my long red nails. I'm told they look very sexual, and the feeling of long nails drawn lightly across a man's back is always very sensual. Women constantly ask me how I manage to look so young. Everyone wonders how I do it, what are my secrets?

Well, there is no magic to it, I'll tell you that. If I can do it, anyone can, and that is why I have written this book.

I am not superwoman. I am a perfectly normal human being. I am still vulnerable to a bag of sweeties or a plate of chips, and when I was drinking wine and champagne I could consume vast quantities without shame or guilt. The same thing with drugs. Yet still I didn't look or feel a wreck, so I figure that amongst the bad things,

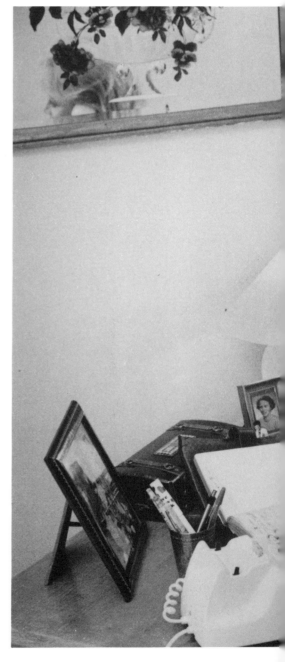

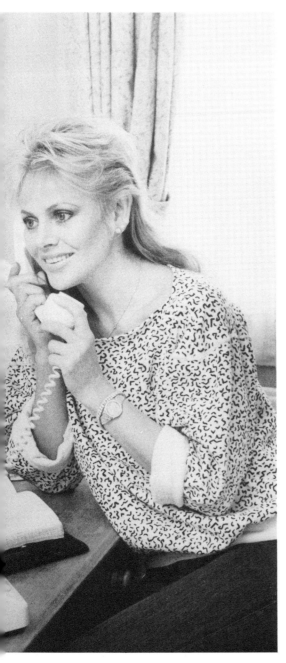

somewhere along the line I am obviously doing it right. I was born with common sense and that is one thing that doesn't desert you.

I am bossy. I admit it. I just can't help telling people how to do things. I say to my friends, 'You don't have to have that pimple' or 'You had a rough night last night, why don't you make some Bieler broth [see p.86] to clean out your liver?' I do feel sad when I see a woman of my age looking as if she is about to step over on to the other side. No one needs to look like that. It is a tragedy. I can't help it, maybe I should have been a nurse.

I believe it is never too late to change. 'Can't' does not exist in my vocabulary. But I don't believe in telling people to deprive themselves of everything they enjoy and I'm not about to tell you to throw your poor, flabby, overweight or underweight, aching body into some horrific, strenuous, superhuman schedule. That is not the Ekland way.

Nor do I suggest you just 'cover up the dark lines under your eyes with this magnificent white stick'. Ultimately you have got to find out why you've got dark circles under your eyes when you sleep fifteen hours a night.

With my usual honesty – and this is a Swedish trait – I want to talk about things that other people don't talk about. I want to go below the surface into that highly complicated piece of machinery we call the body. I want you to get the absolute, 100 per cent best out of it.

There is no miracle involved, no miracle to be paid for. You don't have to be a movie star, a celebrity, a rich woman or born beautiful. Anyone can be born beautiful, but somewhere along the line that beauty fades.

It takes a little time and you need a little solitude. I don't mean physical solitude, I mean mental solitude. You have got to be alone with yourself for a while and not preoccupied with that beautiful handbag in the shop window or tonight's dinner. You've got to look at yourself really hard. Think about what you want to achieve.

Most people automatically say, 'I'll start tomorrow.' If you say 'tomorrow' you have already failed, because there is always another tomorrow. It's got to happen right this minute. Your head has got to say 'today'.

Mine finally did and I am very proud of the little things I have achieved. I want to share them with you.

7

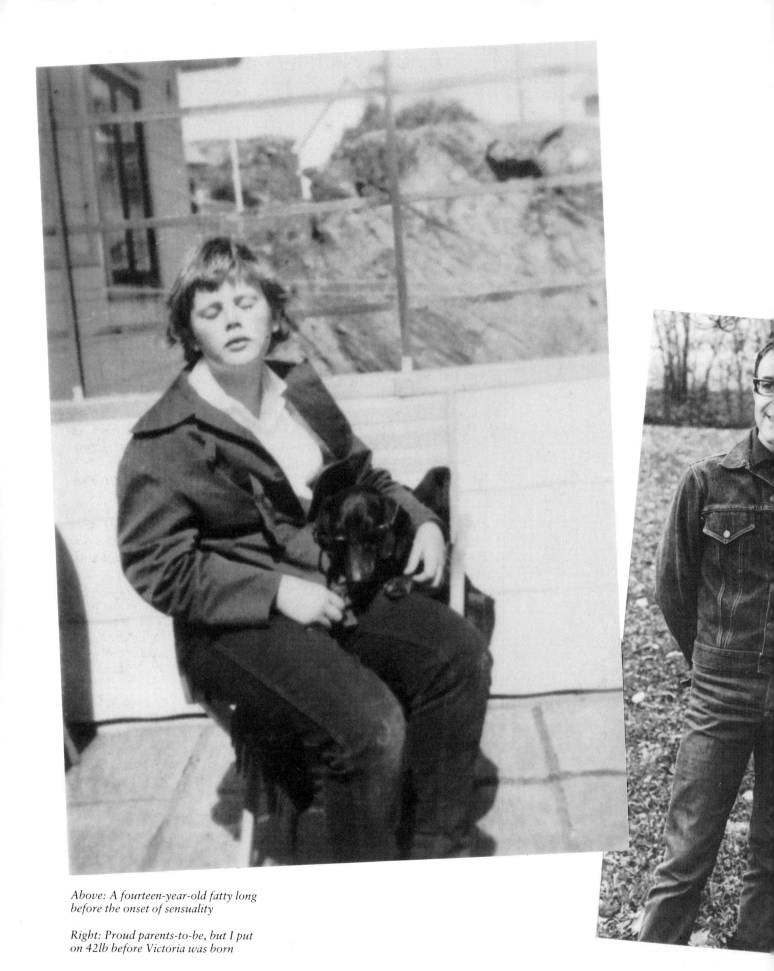

Above: A fourteen-year-old fatty long before the onset of sensuality

Right: Proud parents-to-be, but I put on 42lb before Victoria was born

1/ON BEING BRITT

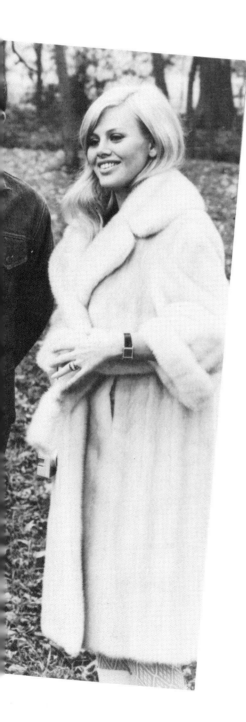

I wasn't born beautiful or rich. I wasn't always the confident, open human being that I am today. 'Fatty' and 'Dumbo' are nicknames not unfamiliar to me.

Sensually speaking, I got off to an inglorious start. When I was a teenager I was imprisoned in a girdle that went from the waist to just below the crutch. Not even a streamlined pantie girdle, but the old kind with suspenders.

In those days, if you were a little overweight, which I was as a child and teenager, you were made to look much like a sausage. First there was this incredibly flat line – no belly, no bum, nothing – then suddenly came a big roll below the crutch and a delightful bulge over the stocking tops.

Imagine my introduction to tights. I was virtually nine months pregnant and living at the Plaza Athénée Hotel in Paris, where Sellers was filming *What's New, Pussycat?*. During the time I carried Victoria I had put on 42lb out of sheer ignorance and unawareness, certainly not out of necessity. I was a blimp, a walking blimp.

The female star of the film was the gorgeous Ursula Andress. One night as Peter and I came into the hotel lobby, Ursula appeared from the lift dressed in her stunning film costume. I know today she probably wouldn't dream of wearing an animal coat, but in those days (January 1964) she did and she was dressed from head to foot in cheetah coat and boots and a cream jersey dress so skin-tight that it looked as if it was glued to her body.

Of course most people in such a garment would have lumps and bumps everywhere. Not Ursula. I stared in amazement and said, 'How did you get it so smooth?' Without warning, right there in the lobby, she pulled up her dress and said, 'Look, tights!'

Nothing has ever been the same since. No hands fumbling at suspenders to get off a stocking. Now hands have to fumble at the waistline to pull the whole blooming lot off!

Those first tights were actually very ugly and, if you recall the mini-skirt era first time around, you will remember them being so short that women regularly revealed the reinforced tops of their tights. Not a pretty sight.

Of course the idea of not wearing a bra and showing your nipples was unthinkable. In those days bras were sewn round and round like ice cream cones. Breasts didn't look like breasts, they were permanent points that looked ready to stab anyone who came too close. I was brought up in an open atmosphere; none of the family really bothered to cover up. But being open isn't sexy and despite my family's approach I grew up knowing nothing, absolutely nothing, about my body or sex.

I'd been grossly overweight from the age of six until my periods came, which was quite late – I was about fifteen. Those years are very important, formative ones and the image you have of yourself then never really leaves you. I was stuck with 'Fatty' and 'Fatso'. Another little delight was being called 'Dumbo' because I was born with my ears sticking out. I also had two very long front teeth, so I looked much like a little rabbit. When I married Sellers I had them filed down and that made a big difference.

My mother always told me confidence-inspiring stories about how, when I was a baby, she would try to pin my ears in by bandaging them tightly to my head. But apparently whenever I moved they would just pop out again. In my early movies, if my hair had to be swept up my ears were pinned down with double-sided sticky tape. You could always count on one ear popping out in the middle of a take, so I've given that up as a bad job and now I insist on having my hair cover them. The true Ekland ears have been hidden in every shot in every movie and in every photograph – until now!

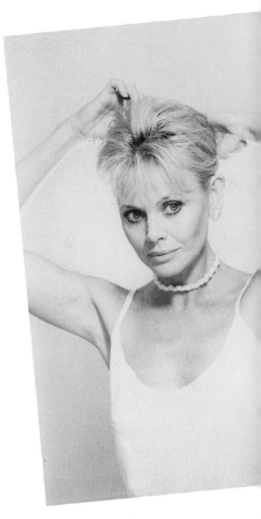

In the 1950s cosmetic surgery was rare, and unthinkable for something so vain and frivolous. Now it would just be 'snip and you're perfect'. I am very 'pro' cosmetic surgery and heaven knows why I've never done anything about getting my ears fixed. I guess I've lived with them so long. Besides, they do give me, when I want, incredibly sharp hearing which can be very useful indeed. My ears are natural trumpets. The reverse side of that coin is that I have to sleep with ear-plugs.

I was naturally bestowed with hair colour that people today glamorously refer to as Swedish blonde, but we called it 'mousey'. It's basically a monotone silver grey which left to itself perked up a bit in summer. Now I have highlights put in to brighten it up.

Swedish winters are very dark and very cold and very long, so not surprisingly the food our parents gave us was geared to keeping us warm and that meant primarily a high-calorie, high-starch content. No thought of diet ever entered into it.

That famous photo of me with the dog (see page 8) marked my fourteenth summer. You don't know which is Britt Ekland, the dog or the thing that held the dog in her lap. That autumn my body decided to make the transition to woman, and with the arrival of my periods some weight dropped off – but not enough.

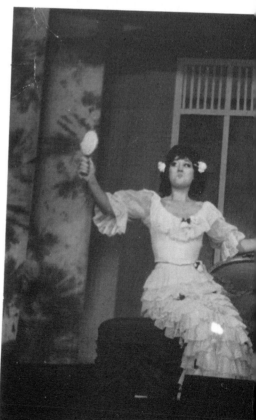

I loathed school and when I was seventeen I escaped into drama school, not just because I wanted to be an actress but also in the hopes of curing me of a common affliction, blushing – though that's too mild a word for the scorching beetroot red my face turned. If the teacher asked me what two plus two was, I wasn't simply shy, my entire body burned. I've been known, even today, to blush when I hear a foul expression or a really dirty joke.

Drama school helped me overcome my shyness but it had one other great plus – it was fashionable to diet and I jumped on the bandwagon. We didn't diet very sensibly, mind you. We would force ourselves to go without food for days on end, then we would succumb to temptation in a major way.

We had wonderful-quality food in Sweden and I would think nothing of tucking away 2-inch slices of marvellous dark bread with great big globs of cheese. Naturally it was not de-fatted.

I think God just helped me along until I was about thirty by now and then putting a thought in my head – cut out the bread, cut out the potatoes, very basic stuff. It's amazing to me that diet books have only really been popular, commonplace items for the last decade.

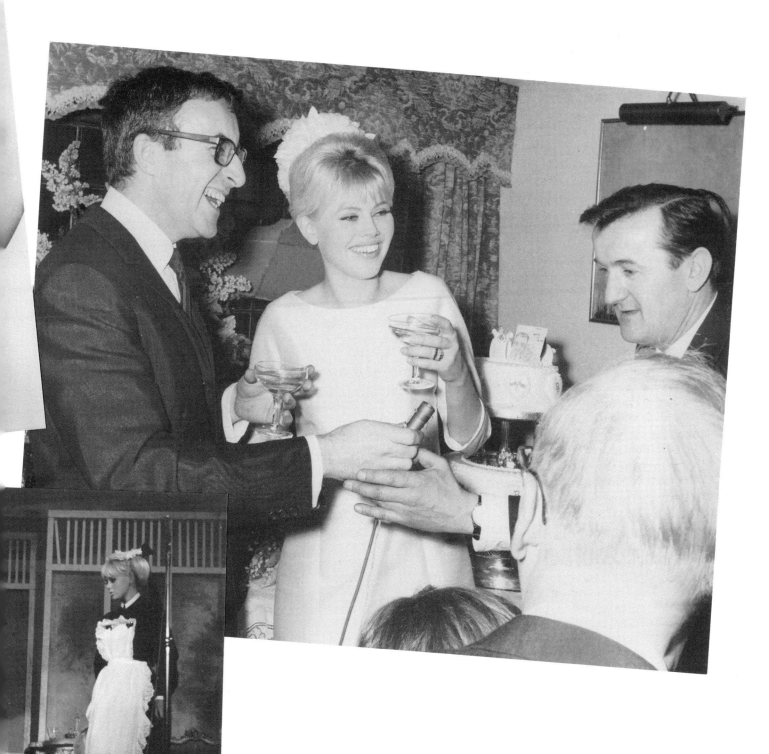

Top left: My 'Dumbo' ears in all their glory – never before revealed on purpose!

Above: My rabbit teeth before capping – my greatest beauty investment

Left: Drama school was supposed to help me beat my blushing

Anyway dieting of one kind or another has been pretty much a way of life for me, on and off, from then until now. I don't understand people who don't have to watch their weight and frankly I'd like to punch them in the face. I can't imagine being able to overeat without suffering the consequences.

I married Sellers at twenty-one and although I'm not pretending the odd physical encounter had not occurred prior to my wedding, I will never forget the horror of finding myself for the first time in close proximity to a man on a twenty-four-hour basis.

How on earth could I deal with going to the bathroom? It wasn't enough to close the door: there was the odd odour to contend with, not to mention having my period. Sellers helped me overcome all that by informing me that he too had once been under the mistaken impression that movie stars and the Queen had it all come ready-wrapped in a neat little cellophane bag.

As far as naughty substances like drugs and alcohol are concerned, I lived a fairly clean life until about 1976. I never was a spirits drinker – it just never appealed to me. When I was about sixteen – way below the legal drinking age in Sweden – I dated a terribly sophisticated gentleman of twenty-one. I'd never set foot inside a bar before, and I'll never forget that first time. The bar was called Cecil's and looked much like a New York cocktail lounge. My companion ordered whisky and soda but yours truly had never tasted a real drink, just the odd sip of wine with my grandparents – since my grandfather was something of a connoisseur – and a taste of beer which I detested. So, at a loss to know what to order, I simply followed my date's lead and said, 'The same as you, please.'

This drink was possibly the most foul thing I'd ever tasted in my entire life. I got drunk as a skunk that night, threw up, and have never, never tasted whisky since. Nor brandy and gin for that matter. I'd be lying if I said I'd never had spirits. Disguised as pretty cocktails like pina colada, I've consumed a few shots. But that's it. I suspect my body is very grateful.

As children we were brought up in a drug-free environment. There may have been drugs in Sweden, but not in our house. I'm not talking about anything sinister either, you understand. When we were really suffering badly with flu and sore throats, my mother might just be pushed into going to the pharmacy. She purchased little packages which today you would probably be arrested for carrying since they looked suspiciously like cocaine. But in fact it was good old aspirin. Just the basic ingredient, not even in pill form. God, this makes me sound a hundred years old! Anyway, the packages opened up like paper ice cream cones and when we were delirious with fever, lying there pouring with sweat, my mother would force this down us. But only in extremis. That was the only drug I took until I was twenty years old.

I truly believe that the fact that thirty of my forty years of life were almost alcohol- and drug-free has helped me enormously. And I don't mean illegal drugs, but prescription drugs too. I took the birth control pill for just five years and never continuously.

After my break-up with Rod Stewart, in desperation I tried anything to numb the pain. I've never taken acid and I've never taken mescaline but I have tried everything else and in all honesty liked it all. But again common sense and vanity and, in recent years, a real awareness of my body, prevented me from being an alcoholic, a druggie and a fat, rolling blob.

My mother was forty-nine years old when she was given five weeks to live, maximum. The weight fell off her right before my eyes. Cancer is a vicious, vicious disease.

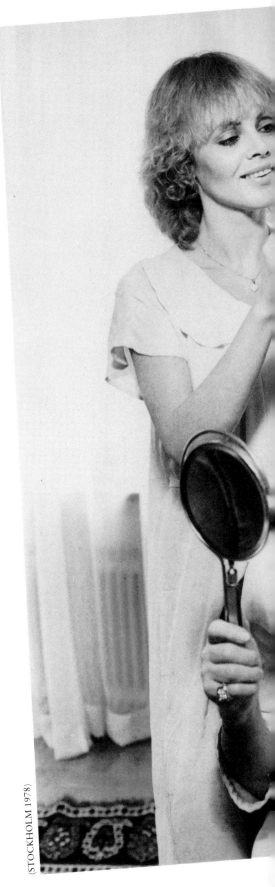

(STOCKHOLM 1978)

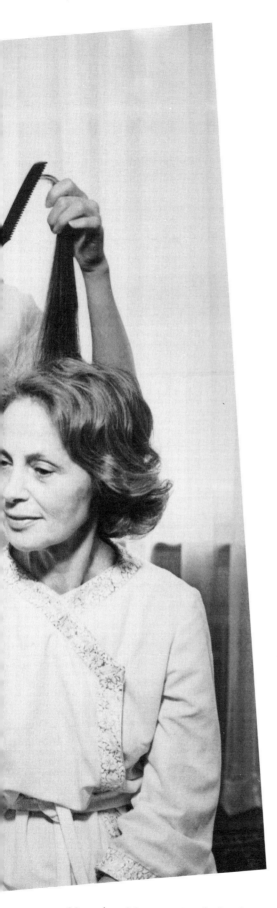

Me and my Mum – notice the family resemblance?

That was fifteen years ago and she survived. Even the doctors think it's a miracle. I was very young when it happened and still married to Sellers, who of course had his own dreadful health problems. I think being close to diseases of two such different types affected me deeply.

Not that I was terrified of having a heart attack. I knew perfectly well that the likelihood of a woman having a heart attack is far, far slighter than the risk for a man. But cancer is a different story. I don't believe it is hereditary. If it runs in a family I think it is coincidence and could have something to do with diet.

Actually, my mother was something of a health freak ahead of her time. She took brewers' yeast and molasses, yet ironically she got cancer and I wanted to know why.

In my mother's case, cancer hit the uterus and female organs. Cancer tends to hit an area that has been traumatized, which is why breasts and female organs are vulnerable in women. Studies on nuns and women who have never had intercourse or given birth bear that out. My mother had given birth to four children and I believe that is why she was physically more vulnerable in that area.

You may think I am totally nuts, but I also believe she was vulnerable mentally. She was probably not aware of it then but she was not a happy person, she was not living a happy life, and I believe that contributed to her getting cancer.

I am convinced that she survived because her previous diet, apart from the meat she ate, had been healthy – no smoking, no drinking, very good-quality pure foods, everything fresh and made from scratch, no processed or tinned stuff. I believe diet is definitely a weapon with which to fight cancer.

She was a very strong woman, a good person through and through, and she lived and she looks beautiful today. But the chemotherapy treatment left its mark and she is no longer strong emotionally or a typical Leo, her birth sign. I believe the family helped her survive. We did not want her to die so we told her that all the time, over and over again.

I had just given birth to Victoria and I kept telling her that I needed her, that she couldn't die because she had a very young grand-daughter to live for.

Some doctors believe that cancer patients die because they are ready to. My mother wasn't ready to die and so she lived.

What finally opened my eyes to my body was the very traumatic upheaval of breaking up with Rod. The break-up of my marriage to Sellers was one thing, but I was younger then, only twenty-five, and I still had the ability to heal easily. It doesn't mean the memories disappeared but the hurt did disappear. With Rod it took a much, much longer time to recover. That is when I started to become totally aware of my body and how what I did with it affected my looks.

I followed the highly inadvisable practice of pigging out and throwing up. Then for a while – and I wouldn't recommend this to anybody in the whole world – I was anorexic. I didn't eat a proper meal from August until the next January. Perhaps once a week I would force down a small piece of chicken and that was it. My emotional troubles threw my body right out of tune.

Luckily my doctor was wise enough to know that you can never force someone to eat. Instead, he gave me a protein drink mixture and in my case my saving grace was being an actress. I knew that if I wanted to survive professionally I would have to pick myself up and look reasonable. So in a sense my vanity helped me.

The protein powder helped my stomach keep producing the correct juices so that I didn't destroy my digestive system. That way, when I

13

was ready to eat I could start. I hadn't done untold damage to my vital organs, or destroyed my menstrual cycle, lost all my hair, dehydrated my skin or developed tremendous wrinkles.

For the first time I was forced to study myself and my body in an intelligent fashion. I finally recognized the fact that for years I'd been giving it conflicting messages: exercising like crazy at Lotte Berke's strenuous class, then rushing home and stuffing my face with cake and bread and cheese, believing, in my divine ignorance, that having exercised I could allow myself to do that. What rubbish! Just because you lift your legs a few times, you cannot put more food into your body. Exercise oxygenates your body, tones it, firms it and basically keeps it in good nick, but it does not give you *carte blanche* to overeat as I did.

I don't believe in harping on the past but I have to admit that it took me a long time to learn from experience. I made the same mistakes again and again – just like women who repeatedly fall in love with the wrong kind of man.

Age comes very fast if you are not looking out for it. People think it creeps up, but that's not true. One day, you're firm, and bang, the next you're flabby. Yesterday smooth, today wrinkles. Age doesn't like to announce itself. Whenever it is, we all face that one day when we have to face ourselves.

Luckily for me the light dawned in time and I changed my life. Some people like to think that I struggle every day to retain my 'youthful figure', my 'beauty'. They think that I am practising tremendous self-denial. This is just not true. I don't find it hard, apart from the occasional battle with food. But that is, I think, a universal struggle.

I don't really drink and I don't miss it. Going to exercise class is not a chore. I love the challenge. Sometimes I miss going for months at a stretch, but that's just a temporary mood change. Then just as suddenly I get back into the swing of it. I would like to dispel the myth that to feel good and look good you have to be in a permanent state of deprivation. Yes, there are days when you have to stop yourself from eating, but to my mind that's a small price to pay.

Tackle your goals a week at a time and don't set them so high that you get discouraged. Don't set yourself six-month projects, take it week by week.

If, for example, you decide to give up drinking, in the beginning your body is bound to crave it still from time to time. So take it one day at a time to start with.

Even if you don't touch another drop, it takes three months for the bloat to go out of your body – that was my experience anyway – so you have to be patient, but the results are well worth it. Set goals you can reach and you won't be disappointed.

I don't feel forty is a dangerous age. I don't feel it is scary and truly I don't feel that it has made any difference whatsoever to my life. Sometimes it makes a difference in the minds of people around you. They think that if you're in pretty good nick you must have been taking youth pills or health cures or have sneaked away in secret and had everything lifted.

I can't believe some of the things that are written about me. Why won't Britt Ekland age gracefully? What ageing are they talking about? My cars grow old and break down, so do my washing-machine and my cooker, but not *me*.

The images people have of me stem mainly from reading about the life I've led, but I've been involved with such extremes that it's hard for people to realize that the person who married very young into a social circle which involved the royal family is the same person who went to the opposite end of the pole with the rock 'n' roll world.

The image that people have of me is that I'm unapproachable, but I think I'm a very approachable human being. A screen image is so enormous that it's always hard to deal with and when people see the real me, they're always surprised about something. I've reacted that way myself when I've met famous people.

Funnily enough, most women like me once they realize I am flesh and blood. They feel totally free to come out with comments like, 'I thought you had much bigger tits' or 'I thought your hair was much darker'.

Because of my reputation and my book, *True Britt*, people feel they have the right to comment on my life, my weight, my having experienced sorrow – and they do. Once you've exposed yourself you really are public property. At parties I can see them weighing me up. I can see the searchlights scouring for facelifts, but generally the comments I get are complimentary.

I'm a very open-minded person and I've led a very, very full and public life, but contrary to the impression the media like to give, I don't consciously go out and seek young lovers. I do, however, find myself drawn to young people. Maybe it's because I've been exercising on and off for the last ten years, maybe because I take the right vitamins, but mentally and physically my energy level certainly matches that of people much younger than I am.

Young people seem drawn to me too. Not long ago when I went to a club in Los Angeles, four young men came up and asked me to dance. It was a big warehouse-type place, nothing swishy or elegant, and all four were probably at least ten to fifteen years younger than me. I asked my friends if it happened because I was Britt Ekland. They said, 'No, they don't know who you are.'

I think young and I believe my mental attitude shows through in my face. Perhaps that is what makes the biggest difference of all between me and a lot of over-forties. I have no intention whatsoever of slowing down or growing old or giving in to anything. Those words aren't part of my vocabulary, nor will they ever be. I'm stronger, happier, more confident, daring, determined and positive than ever. Who could ask for anything more?

I'm putting myself under the microscope in this book and letting you have a look at me, no holds barred. Hopefully, by the end of it, a lot of eyes will be open a little wider and you will trust me enough at least to try the Ekland way.

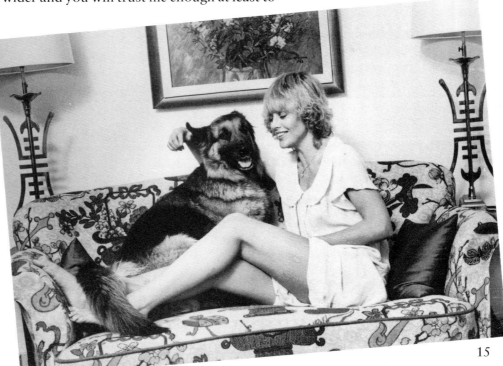

(STOCKHOLM 1978)

15

2/SEE YOURSELF, KNOW YOURSELF

Doing It for Yourself

The single most important statement that you, as a woman, can make is 'I want it for myself.' If you say to yourself, 'I am going to look fabulous', you can do it. If you say to yourself, 'I am going to have a slim, firm body', you can do it. But it has got to be 'me' and 'I', not 'we', 'him', 'her', or 'they'.

If you are changing for someone else, forget it. It won't happen. If your man wants you to lose 10lb, I am sure that if you want to keep him badly enough and that is the ultimatum, you'll probably do it. But if it's not instigated by you and coming from your heart, it won't last.

Maybe you don't want to change and your husband or lover doesn't want you to change. If he likes the way you look, then fine, you shouldn't change.

But I have this horrible, sneaky suspicion that every woman in the world has a little bit of a fright when her husband pats her wobbly middle and says, 'I like you like this, dearie', and that she probably thinks, 'Oh God, if only I could get rid of it.' But as long as he keeps reassuring her, she won't do anything about it and she'll continue to feel dissatisfied with herself. What a waste!

I love Britt Ekland – I think she is a terrific person. That is how I have finally come to feel and I only wish I could have felt like this ten years ago. This is not an ego trip, and it's not narcissism – it's a feeling I have inside and it's so wonderful that I want every woman to share it.

I am confident in myself and my abilities. I please myself without feeling guilty about it. I pay myself compliments. I surround myself with people who make me feel good about myself and with beautiful things. I've learned to love myself. Unfortunately most people don't love themselves. I totally believe the old saying that you can't love someone else properly unless you love yourself first. The more you learn to love yourself, the more you can love your mate.

Of course it's very hard to love yourself when all you do every day is cover up. You cover the bad skin, you cover the bulging belly, you cover the corns, you cover the roots. You can continue covering, of course, but why not stop covering so fast and stand back and examine yourself as you really are?

Don't just wake up in the morning, slap on a bit of make-up and run off to work. Stand naked in front of the mirror and stare hard. If need be, get another mirror to help. Put it between your legs, put it

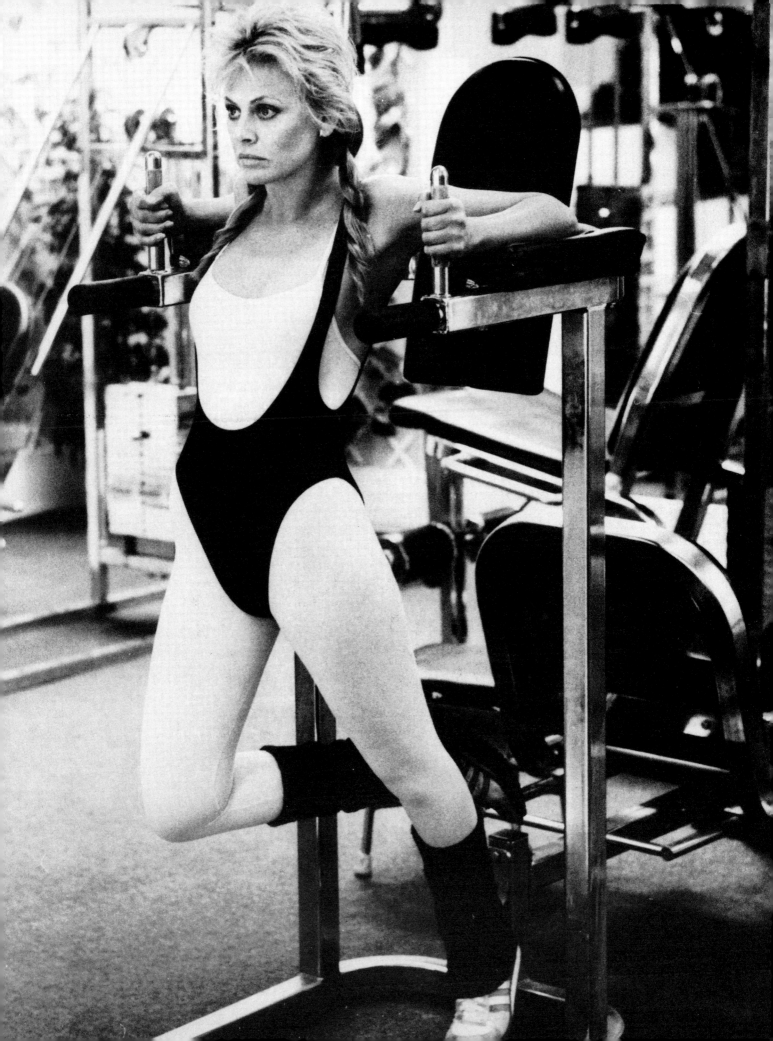

underneath your arms, just look and look and keep on looking. Be disgusted if that's how you really feel, but confront yourself and decide exactly what you would like to change and improve. Believe in your potential and challenge yourself to reach your goals. Once you have made up your mind, *really* made up your mind, the sky's the limit.

Why a Sensual Beauty Book?

Because I believe most women don't feel sensual about themselves and they don't know what they're missing! Since they don't love themselves enough, they don't touch themselves enough. They let other people touch them, but they don't touch themselves and they don't know what they really feel like.

Sensuality is delicious and goes hand in hand with loving yourself. The original, all-time sensual woman to me is Brigitte Bardot. There's no contest. I have never met her, but her entire aura is sensual.

I have always thought Elizabeth Taylor sensual because I believe that, like me, she is vulnerable underneath. She has been called every name under the sun, she has been thin, she has been fat, she has been drunk, she has been sober. To me that proves she is a human being, a woman. She's flesh and blood underneath the image.

Sophia Loren is a timeless beauty but she doesn't move me. She seems untouchable, unreachable, and she doesn't strike me as sensual. Beauty doesn't automatically make a woman sensual, but sensuality makes a woman, any woman, beautiful. I don't care how big, small, fat, skinny, pretty or ugly you are. If you can achieve that feeling of sensuality for yourself, that is all you need to have your own kind of beauty.

Sensuality is subtle and it's something you signal from inside to everyone around you. When you are down, you give out 'down' signals. It doesn't matter how beautiful, how rich or how elegant you are. No one wants you when you give out negatives. When you are up again, suddenly people swarm all round you because they are attracted to your positive signals.

I can hear the sceptics among you saying, 'Good signals, bad signals – it sounds like a load of old mumbo-jumbo to me!' Well, it isn't. The results are real and tangible.

For one thing, if you follow all the advice in this book and raise your awareness of your body and your sensuality, you are bound to have a better sex life. You can read about G-strings and G-spots till the cows come home, but ultimately it comes down to you and your body and being open enough to explore and understand it.

I realize that you may have to take into consideration the minor detail of peeling fifteen potatoes for lunch and putting six kids to bed at night, but I trust that, come the time of day or night or week or month when you hope to make love, you care enough to make sure your legs are waxed and your underarms de-fuzzed.

These are not tasks to perform specifically for sex. They should be a constant part of your routine because you want to be sensual and attractive. The aim is to reach a point where you don't have to creep around and undress in the dark, where you finally love yourself enough to be proud to undress with the bright lights on.

When you are confident, you can play games for fun – go to bed in waterproof mascara or whatever it is – but you don't feel lost without make-up, you don't *have* to do it. You know you are attractive as you are.

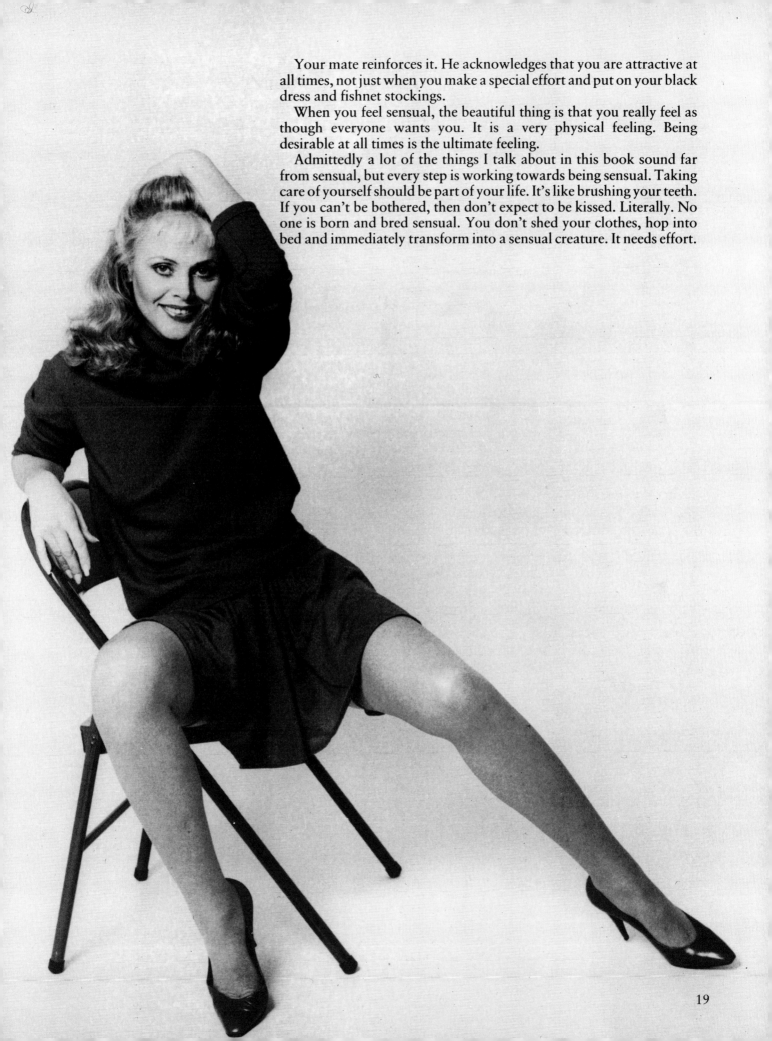

Your mate reinforces it. He acknowledges that you are attractive at all times, not just when you make a special effort and put on your black dress and fishnet stockings.

When you feel sensual, the beautiful thing is that you really feel as though everyone wants you. It is a very physical feeling. Being desirable at all times is the ultimate feeling.

Admittedly a lot of the things I talk about in this book sound far from sensual, but every step is working towards being sensual. Taking care of yourself should be part of your life. It's like brushing your teeth. If you can't be bothered, then don't expect to be kissed. Literally. No one is born and bred sensual. You don't shed your clothes, hop into bed and immediately transform into a sensual creature. It needs effort.

19

3/SKIN CARE: THE SOFT TOUCH

Ultimately the most sensual feeling of all is the feeling of your skin – the touch of skin on skin. Skin is intrinsically sensual, and with a little care you can keep it soft, smooth and young-looking.

If you've got long hair, lift it up and feel the back of your neck. It probably feels as soft as a baby's bottom. Anywhere the sun and wind can't reach is always very lovely. My skin care routine is geared to achieving that kind of softness all over.

Your Body

Keeping Clean

I can't remember a day in the last twenty years when I haven't scrubbed my body hard with a friction mitt. It's an essential part of my daily shower routine and I'm sure that's why my skin stays so soft.

I don't like natural loofahs – they swell to enormous, unmanageable proportions and it's like struggling with a monster from outer space. As a child, my mother used an old-fashioned body brush on me but I prefer a nylon scrub mitt that greatly resembles a Brillo pad in texture.

If you only rinse dirty dishes there's a film left behind and the same goes for your body. What good is it to lay a little soap on top and rinse? You've got to scrub.

I would never use soap on my face, but I soap my body with the mildest brands I can find. Something with the minimum perfume like Neutrogena, Johnson & Johnson or Dove and, as with moisturizer, I switch brands regularly.

I put my hand inside the mitt, lather up with soap and give a good hard rub on knees, heels, soles of feet and backs of hands because they're the ugly bits. If you do this daily, that's all the care they need to keep them smooth and soft. If you've neglected them, keep giving them an extra scrub until they get back into shape.

I also give my bum a good brisk rub, as well my thighs, my stomach, my neck and even my breasts. If I get caught without a mitt then I go through the same routine with a flannel, but I never miss a day's scrub.

If I'm in the mood I switch to a cold shower. I can't call it an everyday occurrence for me because it's bloody uncomfortable, but afterwards you feel nice and tingly and if you use it to rinse off hair conditioner it does make your hair shine. It's good for puffy ankles, too. The one time a cold shower is fabulous is after a sauna – then it makes you feel like a million dollars.

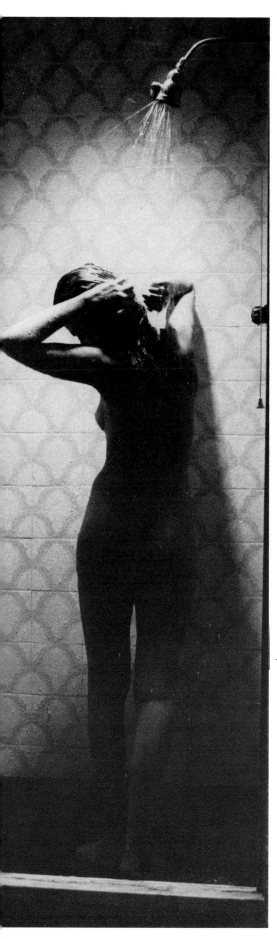

I have a sunken Roman bathtub in my home in Los Angeles but – this sounds very spoilt, and of course I am very spoilt – it takes so long to fill that I never use it. Bathing is a very European habit. Most Americans wouldn't dream of it. I far prefer a shower because in baths I always have the feeling that I'm soaking in my own dirt.

Occasionally I fancy a soak to relax, but I always shower after to get clean. I put pine oil in the bathwater – I love anything pine-smelling – or Masada Dead Sea mineral salts.

I never soak for longer than ten minutes because it dries the skin, and I cut it even shorter if I've got to put make-up on and go out soon afterwards. Baths can make you very red-faced and it takes quite a while to cool down.

* After a night of strenuous sex – or indeed any sex – I recommend that anyone over twenty douches. I know that women in England aren't big on douching but once or twice a week guarantees freshness. It's a particularly good idea after your period to get rid of all the 'debris'.

You don't have to blush when you buy a douche bag in the chemist's – they're quite common. Either use Betadine solution or a large tablespoon of white vinegar with a pint of warm water. Never buy perfumed douches.

Body Lotions and Moisturizers

Contrary to popular belief, the body doesn't end at the chin. Body lotion is vital after every bath or shower, whether you are twelve, twenty, thirty, or forty. Use it on every inch of you.

Unscented lotions that don't clash with your perfume are best for everyday use. I keep Guerlain's Shalimar body lotion for special occasions, but unless something exciting is going to happen to me I wouldn't dream of putting it on my legs because it's terribly expensive. Nivea lotion is good, it's heavy, but you need that in California. Otherwise use any vitamin E-enriched lotion. Don't just smooth on body lotion: literally massage it into your skin, paying special attention to elbows, heels and knees.

Once you've got stretch marks, unfortunately you're stuck with them. If you have a well-trained skin like a gymnast's with a lot of tone you're less likely to get them, but if you're planning to lose weight or

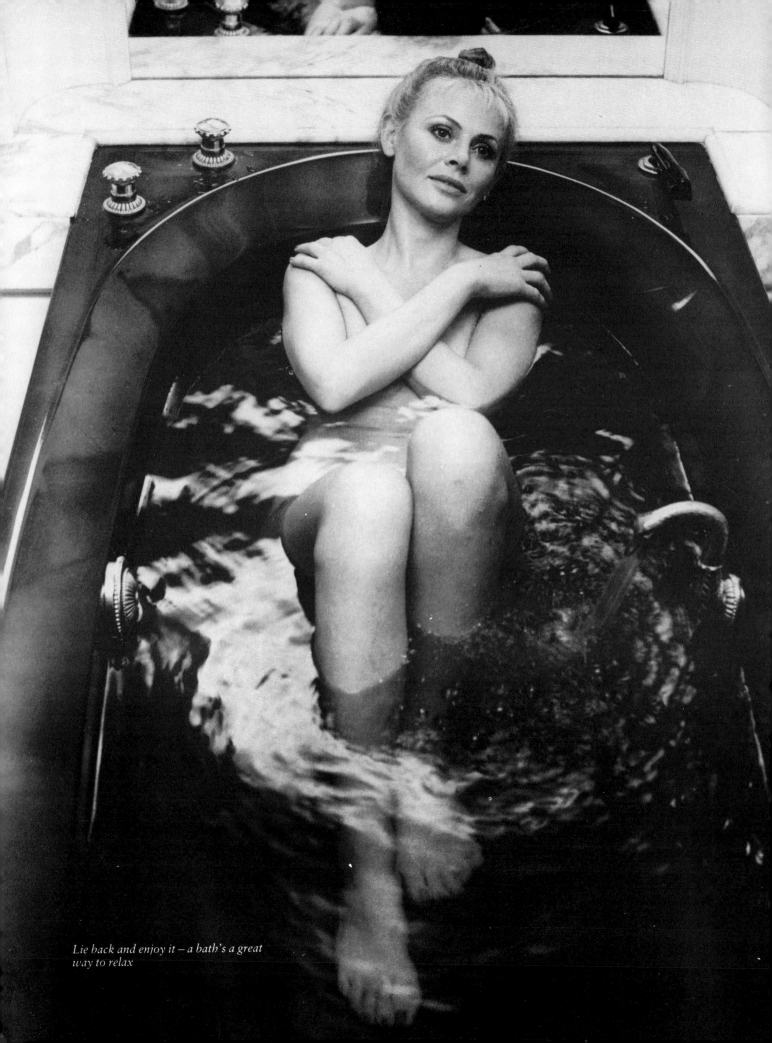

Lie back and enjoy it – a bath's a great way to relax

are pregnant, take the precaution of massaging lots of body lotion around your stomach, breasts, upper arms, thighs, and bottom.

I wouldn't waste money on buying special breast creams but I suggest massaging the cream around your breasts starting under the armpits, circling underneath and up between the breasts. Make five or six circular movements until the lotion sinks in.

You can firm your breasts with exercise – I know, because I've done it. You can't lift them up, but they won't fall down if you keep your pectoral muscles in shape, and no matter how old you are it will make them firmer.

Saunas

Saunas and steam baths are sensual – all that sweat! – and, what's more, they make your skin feel terrific. When I was a child I hated saunas. I could never see the point of sitting in a tiny room sweating, and then rushing out into the snow or jumping into a hole in the ice, which is what my father did.

These days I'm rather partial to a very hot sauna followed by a cold shower, and I can see that they're not just desirable but downright beneficial if you're feeling really dreadful after a festive late night when lots of food and drink have been consumed. A sauna sweats impurities out of your system fast.

I wouldn't recommend a sauna before lovemaking, because you can feel weak and your body continues to sweat for some time. In fact I don't consider going in my sauna unless I can stay home for at least three hours afterwards. I remain in the sauna for a maximum of ten minutes, take a cold shower, and then lie down for twenty minutes.

The heat in the sauna dries out your hair, so it's a good idea to shampoo it, towel dry, and then put on conditioner and pop a shower cap, plastic bag or towel on top. Rinse it off in the shower.

Saunas also dry out your skin. Make sure your face is very clean before you go in, as your pores will open and you will sweat out impurities. After your rest, compensate for the drying effect by giving your face a good helping of moisturizer and treating your body to lashings of body lotion. But wait until you've stopped sweating or it will just pour off again.

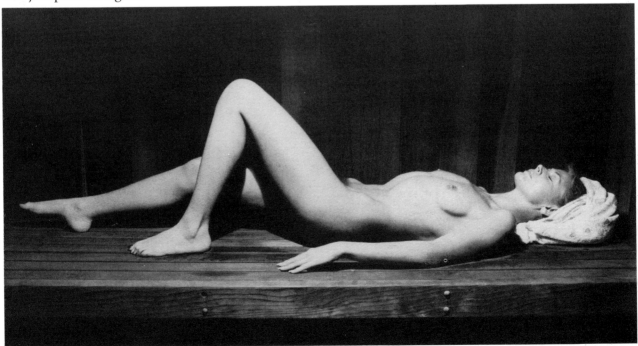

Your Face and Neck

The Cleansing Routine
Men tend to have very good skin beneath their beards – shaving takes off a layer every day. I swear by gritty, skin-sloughing creams which do the same thing. When I am in Los Angeles I have a weekly salon facial, but when I am travelling I give myself the following facial treatment:

1. Cleanse face and neck thoroughly with cleanser.

2. Get a good grainy skin scrub – I use an almond one but there are various types on the market. Take a blob and work it over your face with your fingertips, rubbing quite vigorously on the forehead, between the eyebrows, around the nose and in the chin area. Go gently on your cheeks and very lightly indeed around the eye area, without dragging the skin. Rinse it off with hottish water and you'll find that your skin – minus the grimy top layer – is left fresh and glowing.

3. A face mask comes next. There are a zillion trillion to choose from and I swap around. If my skin is very dry from travelling I will pick a nourishing, moisturizing mask. If I've been in smog-land I choose a deep cleansing one to lift out all the grime that gets lodged in the pores. Sometimes I just want a plain old tightening mask.
   Smooth it on to your face and neck with your fingertips and work it well into the crevices in the chin and around the nostrils, but leave the eye area free in two big, panda-like circles. I try to keep it off my eyebrows because it takes ages to get it off again.

Clarins make a blue gel especially for the eye area but I don't usually bother. Nor do I bother with mashing up avocados or concocting home-made masks. What's the point when it's just as cheap to buy a tube or sachet, and so much simpler?
   If you have puffy eyes, fold a facecloth into a rectangular pad and dip it into ice water. Place the pad across your eyes and, when it warms, dip it back in the ice water. Repeat a few times.
   Tea bags are also effective. Used ones are fine, either camomile or just ordinary tea. Squeeze the bags out, put them in the freezer compartment for ten minutes, then plonk them on your eyes. You'll look like a new woman. Or dip cotton wool pads into ice-cold camomile tea.
   I have a strange-looking alternative. I call it my Lone Ranger mask because that's what it looks like and it gives everyone a good laugh at the breakfast table. It's filled with a soothing, cooling blue liquid that takes down any puffiness and you keep it in the fridge so it is permanently chilled. Mine was a birthday gift bought in the U.S.A. but there are various brands including European Aqua-Pac, Looky and Masque de Gelé.

Moisturizers
When I step out of my morning shower I wrap up my hair in a towel, and while my skin is still warm I break open a collagen ampoule. I use Formule Équilibrante Ampoules Visage by Sothys of Paris – they're expensive little glass vials, but I do find the formula really makes my skin look glowing and translucent. Our skin's collagen production slows down as we get older, causing sagging and wrinkles, and collagen ampoules are meant to help keep those effects at bay.
   Since my skin gets so much wear and tear when I'm working, I splash out and use them every day, regardless of what it says on the

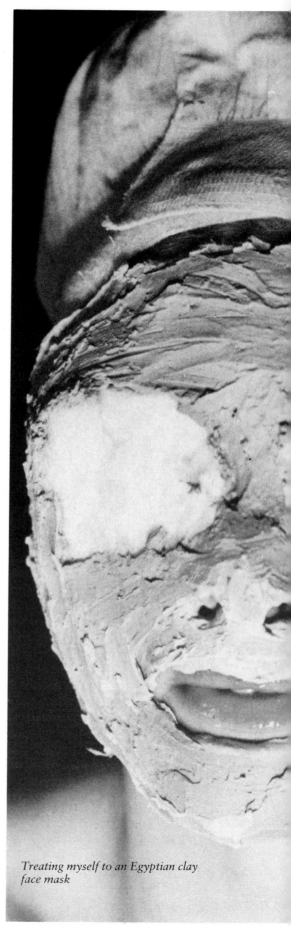

Treating myself to an Egyptian clay face mask

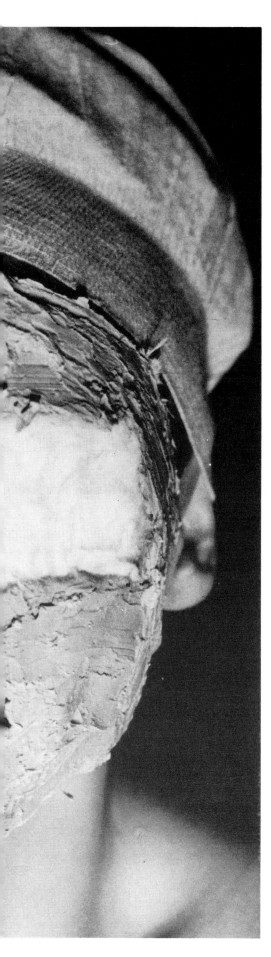

package. I pat the contents of the ampoule all over my face and neck and let it sink in, especially round the eye area. I work it in with light stroking movements – up strokes on the face, down strokes on the neck.

By the same token, I do treat myself to expensive eye creams and anti-wrinkle creams if I believe in them – after all, my face is my fortune.

I use La Prairie Eye Contour Cream morning and night. The La Prairie products are Swiss and yes, they're expensive, but they're worth it in my opinion and they last for ages. The delicate skin around the eyes is especially prone to wrinkles, and a good eye cream can do a lot to combat loss of moisture and keep them at bay. I don't think that you can ever put enough moisturizer around your eyes. I sometimes use La Prairie Cellular Wrinkle Cream on top of the eye cream too, during the day as well as at night.

Cheaper alternatives to use around your eyes are a simple vitamin E stick or good old almond oil.

Anti-wrinkle formulas should only be used on the areas that are prone to wrinkles. Put them on between your eyebrows, all the way around your eyes, down the crease lines from your nose to the corners of your mouth, and all the way around your mouth – not on your mouth but just outside the lipline. And always pat the cream in with light movements.

I believe in swopping creams every month or so and my alternative choice is Unibiogen Juvena Exclusives, another Swiss range that is absolutely superb. I will use the Highly Active Unibiogen Concentrate – an oil which I am assured will last at least a year – for a month, then go back to La Prairie Wrinkle Cream.

I make a beeline for manufacturer's trial sizes or products with a free offer attached. That's a cheap way to find things you like and once the little jars are empty I use them in my travel kit.

I change daytime moisturizers regularly and find my skin responds well. Swopping creams is a bit like suddenly taking care of your skin after a period of neglect – one minute it's dry and prune-like, a week later it looks distinctly improved.

If my face is constantly being photographed and I'm sitting under hot lights, covered in fairly thick make-up, from seven in the morning until late at night, I once again favour an expensive cream like Juvena's Unibiogen Moisture Balance or La Prairie. Quite frankly, my skin needs it. But if you're just going to wear a light make-up and live in the country where the air is fresh, you don't really need it.

I believe there are plenty of good, cheap products around. I often use a simple Vitamin E moisturizer like Cabot's or a very pure product like Rachel Perry's Moisture Cream which you can buy in health food stores. Another moisturizer I like is Nivea. Don't be afraid of using it just because it's cheap.

It goes without saying that every time you moisturize your face you should moisturize your neck too. Putting cream on your face and ignoring your neck is, to me, like brushing your top teeth and not your bottom ones. Your neck needs every bit of moisture it can get to keep it smooth and sensual.

Take climate into account when you buy face creams. What might suit you very nicely in England may be totally insufficient in extreme heat. My skin is always at its best in London because of the moisture in the air. Dry, heated hotel rooms are much the same the world over and play havoc with my skin, making it incredibly thirsty. Both the La Prairie creams and Juvena's Unibiogen seem to be just as effective wherever I am in the world.

At night I use Estée Lauder's Cellular Night Repair. It comes with a dropper and you put a drop on forehead, cheeks, chin and neck and then follow it up with night cream. I've found it very effective – it makes my skin positively glow.

Whenever you decide to treat yourself to an expensive product like a collagen cream, do check the label before you buy to make sure that collagen is, if not the first ingredient listed, at least in the top four. That way you know you are getting what you pay for. If collagen is the eleventh ingredient listed you're lucky if the manufacturers did more than wave it over the pot. The same applies to all beauty products – vitamin E cream, for example.

Facial Massage

If you treat yourself to a salon facial it will always include some kind of facial massage. There are various types but they all share the common goal of smoothing away lines and wrinkles and counteracting the downward tug of tiredness and depression. Upward strokes are the keynote.

As with body massage, after you've sampled a few facials you can easily pick up the simple movements and incorporate them into your own routine. Upwards and outwards strokes, for instance – copy them to work in your cleanser, to apply your face mask and, more important still, every time you put on moisturizer. As with your body lotion, the massage movements encourage better absorption of the creams.

Out, Damned Spot!

If you are over twenty-one and you get a pimple, it is probably the result of some unspeakable act of oral gratification, since your diet reflects itself in your face. Ours is not to question why, ours is just to deal with.

Now I know your fingers itch when that little mountain gets a head on it, but you can't tamper with it without running the risk of permanent scarring.

A salon face massage is a great skin reviver

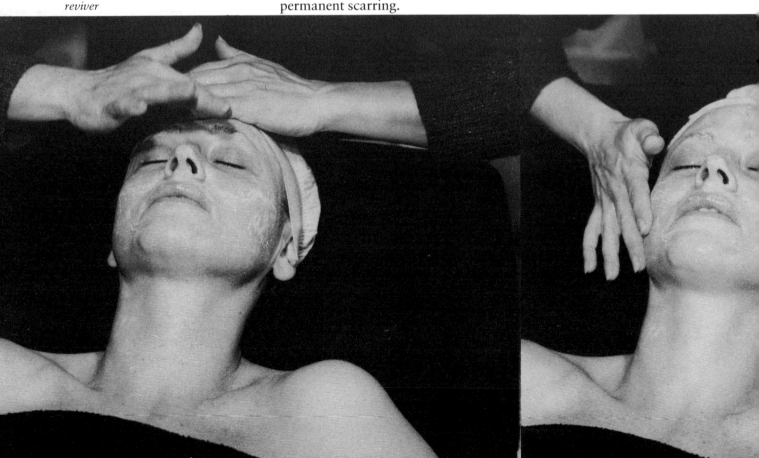

Try preparations containing salicylic acid (which degreases) or benzoyl peroxide (which unplugs the pore) to get rid of stubborn pimples fast. If you don't have either handy, dab alcohol or perfume directly on to the spot with a pristine clean finger. The drying properties will help. Never put any cream on it – the whole object is to dry it out as much as possible.

If spots are a recurring problem, I'd recommend you to have facial treatments at a salon where they may use a steamer to help clear out your pores, and that's not something I think you should ever attempt at home.

Liplines

Those little lines above the top lip come from smoking or pouting, and in my case it must have been pouting – if one was a sex symbol one was supposed to pout.

When we were children my mother had the foresight to give us some protection – she wouldn't let us go out in the cold without moisturizer and lip salve. Today I am just as fussy, even if I am just sitting in a centrally heated room.

I always carry a vitamin E stick and circle it round my eyes and then round my lips. If you are prone to liplines, carry the stick beyond your natural lipline.

Ears

These are a much neglected piece of our anatomy. Use cotton buds whenever you wash your hair or get water in your ears. I clean my ears every day because everyone's ears tend to look a little greasy inside, and if you whisk a cotton bud round all the little crevices you can get rid of it.

Traditionally the prime site for perfume has been behind the ears, but go easy on it. If someone is whispering sweet nothings to you, you don't want them to back away because the smell is too strong. Just because you like the perfume doesn't mean that he will!

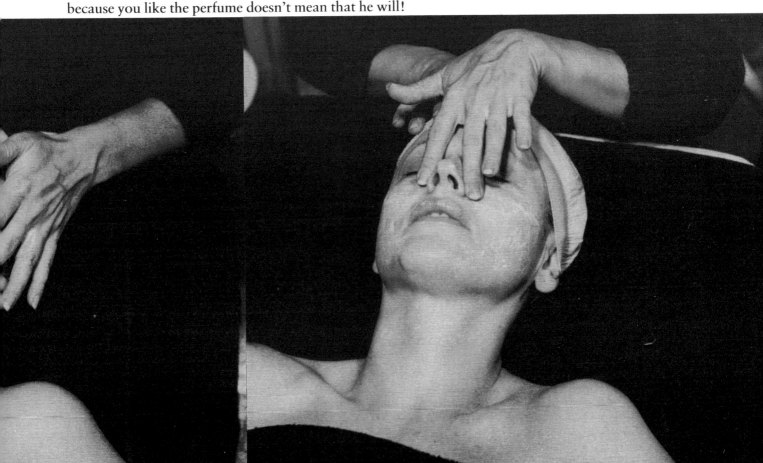

Taking a Tanning

OK, I confess. I used to be a sun addict. I learned a little too late, unfortunately, that the sun is your skin's worst enemy. This simple statement of fact, however, does not deter 98 per cent of the female population from frying their skin and it did not deter me.

Even in school we kids would fight for the desks closest to the window. Between the hours of eleven and three the victors would assume a strange, angled pose in order to expose as much flesh as possible to the sunlight streaming in through the open windows. The trick was to look utterly nonchalant and, of course, as though you were hanging on the teacher's every word.

I grew up believing that dark skin is prettier than fair. Things have changed now, but in those days Sweden was very much for Swedes only. There was so much blonde that the effect was completely bland. I think I was eighteen before I ever saw a black person.

We didn't use any kind of suntan lotion and my skin was very white in those days, yet we didn't burn. I am sure the Swedish sun is far less ferocious than it is in say Hawaii, the Bahamas, or even California, where I moved in 1974. California is the suntan state. Everyone is blonde and beautiful with blue, blue eyes and lots of white, white teeth. Californians just glow and that is how everyone wants to look – I did too.

Tanning is inevitable in a sunny climate – you tend to sit outside to do your chores and walk about in next to nothing, but people who live in the sun don't need to indulge in as much concentrated tanning as say Mrs Britain, who goes for her annual four weeks' burn-up – two weeks' deep frying time in the summer and, if she can afford it, two weeks' deep frying time in the Bahamas in the winter.

If you want the best possible all-over tan, watch children. They don't lie glued to a lounger methodically turning themselves every twenty minutes like a chicken roasting in the oven. They put on their bathing suits and jump and run and go boating and swimming, and all that movement truly is the secret of a perfect tan.

The world is full of tanning disaster stories. My problem was an outbreak of ugly brown pigmentation spots everywhere. A lot of women don't realize that if you take the birth control pill you shouldn't venture out in the sun too much. You develop what I can best describe as birthmarks, and they usually crop up across the brow and forehead, round the cheeks and in a delightful little moustache. They're a dead giveaway for telling who takes the pill. The patches are actually melanin pigmentation and it took me close to a year to get rid of them – I went crazy trying to cover them up with make-up. A dermatologist can prescribe an effective cream bleach – I used it successfully on my chest and hands. You can also literally purify the patches away by thoroughly cleansing your body and sticking to a pure, healthy diet for about a year.

It's hard to stay completely pale in sunny California and tanned legs and arms look pretty in clothes, but at this point in my life I intend to keep my face and chest well out of the sun. These are the tanning rules I live by.

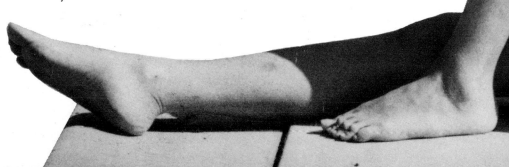

Dos and Don'ts in the Sun

1. Do wear something protective on your skin whenever you go in the sun, even if you're just walking around shopping. Nothing looks worse than sun-parched lips and wrinkly, squinty eyes, and the rays are still beating down on you when you're not sunbathing.

Use a good suntan lotion with a sun protection factor of between 5 and 8 – they are graded upwards according to the amount of burning rays that they block out. If you want to block the sun completely, Bain De Soleil, Ultra Sun Block Creme, sun protection factor 15, does the trick. I've skied with it and sat in the African sun with it, and it hasn't let the sun through.

PABA is an excellent sunblock, especially if you have a sensitive skin like mine. It's a B vitamin – its full name is para-aminobenzoic acid – and is used in various brands of sunscreen. Look for one that puts PABA first in the list of ingredients so that you know it is the predominant component.

PABA acts as a complete block, so if you want to get a tan I suggest you use it on the vulnerable bits as a supplement to your regular suntan lotion. Use PABA on your nose and round your eyes like sunglasses, extending as far as the lines that appear when you squint your eyes in the sun. Don't forget your eyelids and lips – extend it beyond your natural lipline – because they are very prone to sunburn.

2. Do take a multi-vitamin with a high D content to help keep your skin in tip-top shape.

3. Don't ever wear perfume in the sun and that includes spritzing yourself with cologne. Perfume and sun don't agree. The result? Those ugly little brown spots. The same warning applies to perfumed underarm deodorant, moisturizer or body lotion.

4. Don't drink alcohol. I know it's hard to lie there and resist a pina colada with a little umbrella poking out of it, but believe me, alcohol and the sun are a very disagreeable combination. Alcohol dehydrates your body and, since the sun does the same thing, why subject your body to a double dose of bad treatment?

5. Do protect the 'V' above your breasts. You must have noticed how the skin there burns faster. That's because it's as thin as rice paper and once you destroy it by overtanning, there is no cosmetic surgery in the

1975: Still a fearless sun worshipper

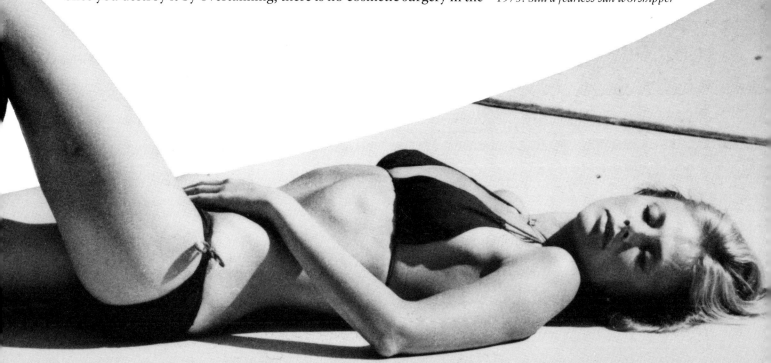

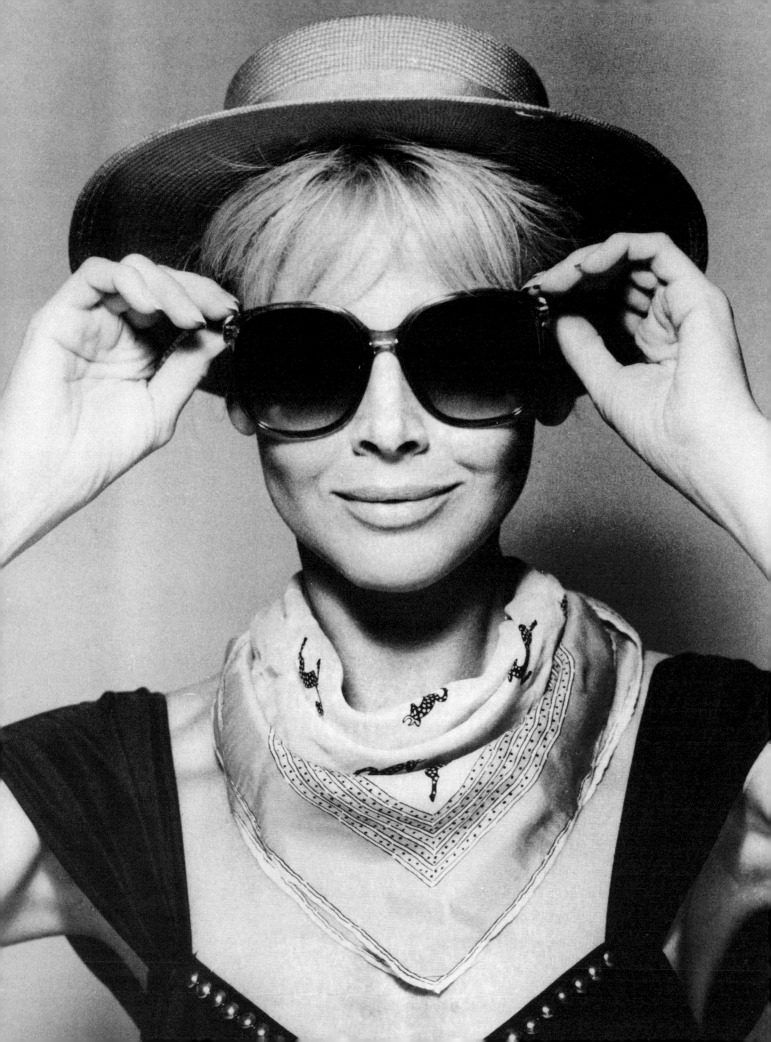

world that can repair it. The best trick I know is to wear a kerchief round your neck. It even looks OK with a bikini, and believe me, it's worth it.

6. Do test out new products before you use them in the sun. This goes for powder, body lotions, suntan lotions, mascara, the lot. Put them in the crease of your elbow before you go to bed – you can test a lot on the same night – and if your skin is clear the next morning you know you're not allergic.

You would think tanning would be a piece of cake for my daughter Victoria, who has a very olive skin. But no. She went to Palm Springs in California and phoned me in tears saying that she had boils all over her face. It turned out she was allergic to the tanning cream she'd used.

You will soon find out if you are allergic to a sunblock or if it simply doesn't agree with you – your eyes will stream and your skin will burn and tingle.

7. Do invest in a straw sunhat and some decent sunglasses to put your face in the shade. Even if you decide to tan your body, save your face.

8. Do use plenty of moisturizer on both face and body. Moisturizing your skin helps prevent peeling and is the only way to camouflage sun-dried skin. If you've somehow managed to get a red, burned nose, try to cover it with make-up, unless it's peeling in which case that will make matters worse. Just keep on moisturizing and, if you need to tone down the redness, try blending in a dab of liquid make-up on top of the moisturizer.

Faking It
If you don't have the time or the sun available to get a tan, and can afford to splash out, I'd definitely recommend salon tanning treatments. The Uvasun system is the best since it's the only one with no harmful UVB rays, which supposedly means you can get a tan without the ageing effects of the sun itself.

If you are going to the beach for the first time, or are going to a party and your legs are white and unattractive-looking, try Sudden Tan for instant results. It's a white cream that creates a tanned effect in a matter of hours, and if you apply it properly it can look very effective.

Make sure your legs are smooth with no bits of hair sticking out. Give them a good scrub and dry them. Smooth on one coat of Sudden Tan as carefully as if you were applying face make-up. Apply it lightly on knees and toe joints and heels – anywhere that the skin is tougher. Bend your knees and toes, too, to make sure you work it into the crevices. I would also try to end the cream in a nice bikini-shape line so that if you find a marvellous date you don't look all straggly round the tops of your legs.

Wash your hands immediately or your palms will turn carrot yellow. Wait for about five minutes until the cream sinks in, then apply a second coat, but steer clear of knees and heels this time. Wash your hands again and wait for an hour to see how the tan comes up. You can always add more if you need to.

I've used it many times and think it is excellent, but I don't care much for its distinctive smell. Still, you have to pay a price for everything! You can use it on your face and body, but if you want to look tanned all over enlist someone's help to blend the cream in properly – otherwise you might end up with a streaky back.

And did you know that you can bring out the pigment in your skin without going anywhere near the sun? Try drinking a big glass of carrot juice, with a squeeze of lemon juice to taste, every morning for four to six weeks.

31

Being a Smoothie

I am fanatical about de-fuzzing. To me there is nothing uglier than seeing a woman in exercise class with a pretty purple leotard, flesh-colour tights, and big bushes sprouting out round her bikini line.

I know there is a school of thought that says men find underarm hair a big turn-on, but to me it's gruesome. God may have made us that way, but he also made man invent razors, so I guess he had second thoughts.

I'm blonde so I don't have a moustache problem, but my daughter Victoria is very dark and so is my mother. My mother bleaches, Victoria waxes – frankly I don't think it matters which method you choose as long as you do it. It is fatal to shave unless your ambition is to grow a beautiful, long moustache and twirl the ends up.

If *you* can see your body hair, you can bet your life other people notice it too. I know the sun lightens dark hair on arms and it doesn't show as much if you're tanned, but unless you're incredibly fond of it, get rid of it. Bleach it if it's a relatively small amount, but if it's a heavy growth you'd be better off waxing.

I know people who shall remain nameless (and therefore shall remain friends) who have straggly hairs growing around their nipples that bear a striking resemblance to pubic hairs. Snip them off – it's safer than tweezing because breasts are a delicate item.

I like my nose, but I don't know why God gave us all this hair in the nostrils. I know it's a filtering system but I wish he hadn't done it – particularly as on film it is magnified to forest proportions. I used to tweeze out stray hairs but woke one morning to a shiny, red hooter three times its normal size. My doctor was mortified. He prescribed large doses of antibiotics and lectured me on the dangers of such foolish behaviour. Apparently there is one nerve in your nose that goes straight to the brain, and tampering with it, as any karate expert will tell you, can kill. Needless to say, I abandoned the habit immediately.

My eyebrows are naturally rather fine and I've never had to tweeze them, but believe it or not I actually tweezed my eyelashes in the sixties – whipping out two or three from the top and bottom was meant to give you a wide-eyed look. Even by my standards it was a stupid thing to do. Well-shaped brows, however, are important and I definitely believe in tweezing out any straggly hairs below the natural browline to neaten up the shape. Slant-edge tweezers are the most efficient. Always tweeze hairs out in the direction of their growth – if you pull against the root they'll grow back crooked. Although fashions in eyebrows come and go, I'd stick to the shape you were born with and confine your tweezing to stragglers only. Once brows are over-plucked they rarely grow back properly. Take your time and make sure that you tweeze equally on each side to keep your brows balanced.

In spite of being blonde I shave under my arms daily. I also shave around my bikini line, summer and winter, every single day. I wouldn't wax there, because it seems a waste of money. I just whisk over with a simple Bic razor and throw it away every week.

My legs are a different matter – they're always on show. It's not that I imagine hundreds of hands grabbing for them every five minutes, but rather that shaved hair grows back stubbly and fast. I don't care how pretty they look in the morning, by the afternoon they're sprouting hair again, so I have them waxed every four to six weeks. (Waxing weakens the hair.) Although there are home waxing kits on the market, I'd always opt for having it done in the salon by a professional. Besides, it's a very messy business. I've tried hot wax, cold wax, wax strips, you name it – and it's just not worth it.

* If your pubic hairs are too long and bushy, take them like a ponytail and with a pair of nail scissors, trim the excess off.

Showing a leg, with no stubble in sight!

32

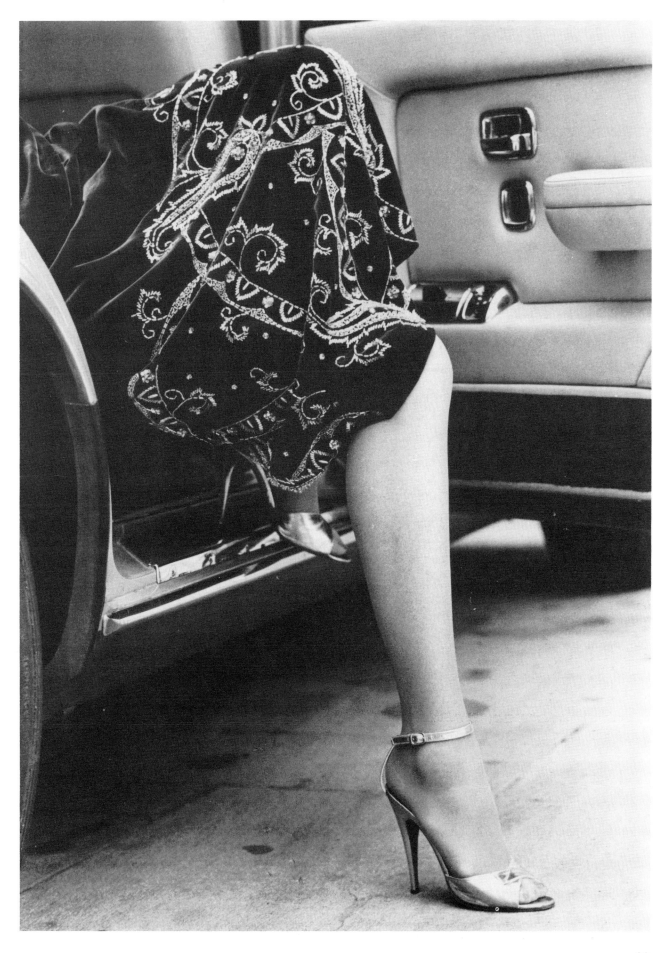

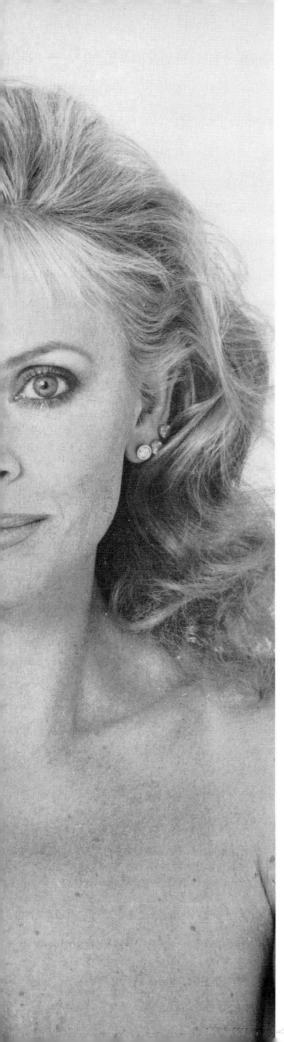

The Long and the Short of It

Queen Guinevere and Lady Godiva knew a thing or two. Hair is a woman's greatest asset, and the longer and silkier the better, in my opinion.

It's a bit of a cliché to say that men love to run their fingers through it, but like all good clichés it's grounded in truth. More important still, *I* love to run my fingers through it. I like the feeling of hair and I like to see it around me. Hairdressers will hate me for saying it, but I'd honestly take long, limp fine hair over short, thick hair any day.

Long hair is sexy, long hair is sensual, long hair is versatile, and I think long hair is the most flattering to most women. It can also hide a multitude of sins like double chins, scars, big ears, and pimply foreheads. My hair is baby-fine, but I like it best of all when it's long and that's how I intend to keep it.

Joan Collins has had her fiftieth birthday but she wears styles that suit her age, make her look youthful, and yet still look as though they are long. What it amounts to is a much more artificial hairstyle if you like – proper set, proper style, much neater.

When I chopped my hair off short I found it changed my mentality. Suddenly I was thinking like a man, and I just didn't feel very feminine. But short hair does feel very free. It may not be particularly sensual, but it's obviously a godsend if you're a very sporty type. It's marvellous to be able to jump in the shower and then just fluff it out. When my hair was cropped I had all the tips bleached snow white and I looked like a porcupine, which was quite fun.

What you can do if you have short hair and still want to look and feel feminine and sensual is wear lots of earrings and necklaces. If you can afford it you could also invest in a half-wig – it's got to be superb quality otherwise it's better not to bother. Mine is like half a bathing cap and hides all my hair except for the front. It comes to the top of the crown, where I pin it in place and then backcomb my own front hair back over it to hide the join. I wore it for about two years while waiting for my hair to grow out before anyone realized that it wasn't my own hair.

If you are overweight, the worst thing you can do is cut your hair above chin-level. The most flattering styles are feathered on to the face – to where your cheekbones would be if they were visible – and feathered around your neck to slim it down.

I don't care how old you are, unless you've got Mia Farrow's or

OF HAIR

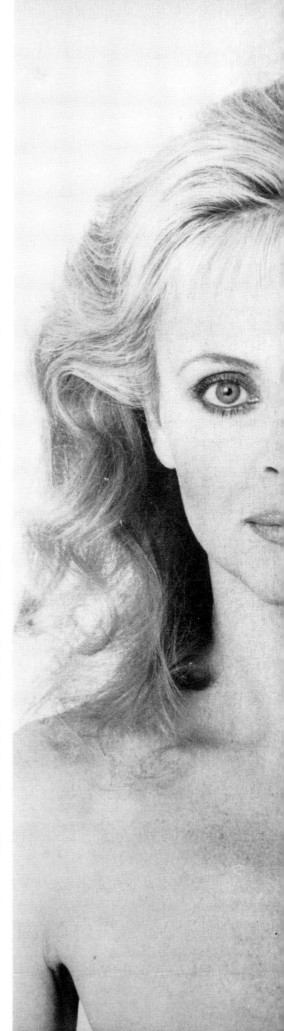

Audrey Hepburn's looks cutting your hair very short simply reveals your double chins in all their glory.

If your face is slim but your body is big, you still need plenty of hair to balance the rest of you. You should always be wider at the top than at the bottom.

What is always sensual is soft, clean-smelling hair. I've found that men aren't very fond of strong-smelling shampoos and naturally a woman should never go to bed with any nets or rollers or other hair implements. Heaven forbid! Freshly washed hair is sensual, even if it's short and fluffy rather than long and silky.

Putting a Good Clean Shine on It

There are approximately 120,000 hairs on your head and in the natural course of events you lose between fifty and eighty a day. Hair is made up of protein and each individual strand has its own 'acid mantle', which is like a protective coating. This coating has a natural acid/alkaline balance and if it's disturbed the hair is damaged and becomes out of condition. In the old days our grandmothers followed a soapy shampoo with a vinegar or lemon rinse – now hair products are sold with built-in pH balance, which means that chemists have worked out the correct balance between alkaline cleansing ingredients and acid factors that return your hair to 'normal'.

Shampoos, like face creams, are very personal. Even with my normal hair some products make it dry, some make it limp, while some make it frizzy. It's trial and error unfortunately but Vidal Sassoon's entire range for sensitive hair is an excellent buy and I absolutely refuse to waste money on anything more expensive. As with moisturizers, I switch shampoos from time to time when they start to become less effective.

I wash my hair in the shower every single day because clean hair makes me feel good and it's a fallacy that frequent shampooing uses up all your hair's natural oils. Since I don't have a week's build-up of grease and dirt to contend with, one lather is sufficient. If you can bear it, a cold water rinse makes it shine.

Whatever your hair type, I don't believe in shampoos with built-in conditioners. Taking dirt out and putting conditioner in is a difficult process and I find that you can wash and rinse forever but your hair just doesn't feel clean. I recommend that you always use a two-step routine of shampoo, then conditioner.

Cream Rinse or Conditioner?

My son can't understand why I don't want him to use conditioner when his Mummy and Daddy use it. Well, Daddy has wonderful, curly, jet black hair and conditioner helps control it. Mummy uses it because her hair is bleached and streaked and permed and needs the moisture. But as I keep telling Nicholai, if your hair is in its natural, unadulterated state you don't need to feed it.

If you've got long hair, a cream rinse – which is really an instant conditioner – makes combing easier and does leave hair looking shiny. Because there is less tangling, there is also less chance of you getting split ends.

If your hair, like mine, is damaged by perming or tinting or hairspray or backcombing or is just plain dry, choose a proper conditioner and leave it on for the prescribed amount of time to do its job before you rinse it off. If you want to be naughty with your hair that's fine, but compensate with tender loving care afterwards.

Either way, don't use too much, and if your hair is oily at the roots give them a miss altogether. Be sure to rinse well.

Monthly Conditioning Treat

If your hair is dry and damaged, use a protein pack; if you just want shine and your hair is basically in good nick, a cream rinse will do. The same method applies either way. Put the conditioner on to your clean, wet hair. Cover your head and hair with a plastic bag, twirl the ends of the bag and pin them to your head so that the conditioner doesn't drip down your neck. When it's secure, top the bag with a woolly hat, since heat is supposed to help the conditioner penetrate better.

I find this method far more efficient than the traditional suggestion that you wrap your head in hot towels. By the time you have heated a towel and wrung it out, it's cold again. Pointless!

Hair Care in the Sun

If your hair is tinted it's important to protect it from the sun. Until recently I was terribly careless in the name of the California look of flowing blonde hair. I'd literally leap into the pool without a second thought and anything wonderful I'd done to my hair at vast expense would, of course, instantly turn either delicate green or brassy yellow.

Today I know better. I always put conditioner on my hair before sitting outside. There are plenty of special conditioners for sun protection, but any one will do. I put it straight on my hair without wetting it and then tie the lot up in a scarf. There are pretty ways to tie scarves, so you don't need to look like a washerwoman, and it's worth the effort. What's more, you are giving your hair a conditioning treat into the bargain.

Putting in the Style

It's a complete waste of precious time to set your hair, in my opinion. It might have been fine for our mothers who, heaven knows why, only washed their hair once a week. I vividly remember putting gallons of talc into my greasy hair, and can't imagine why when it would have been so much simpler just to wash it.

These days I don't have the time or inclination for anything fussy. The best way to get body into your hair is to bend right over and brush

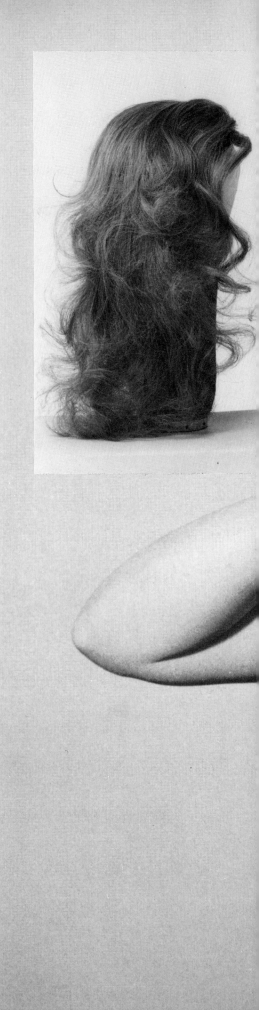

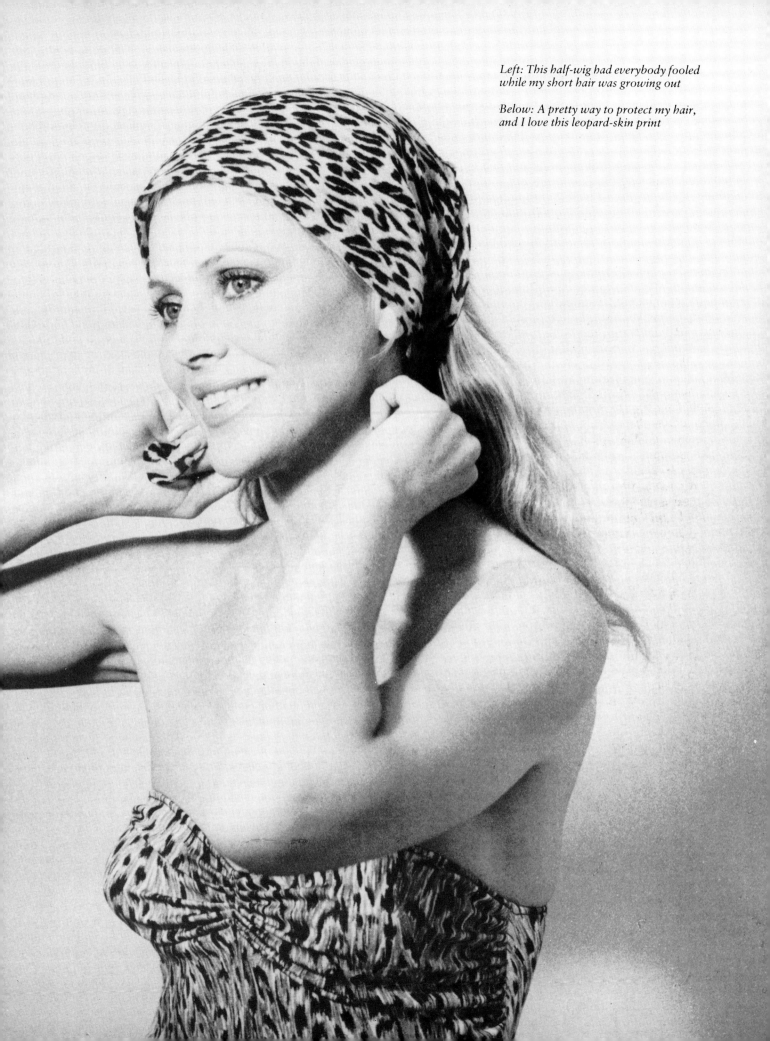

Left: This half-wig had everybody fooled while my short hair was growing out

Below: A pretty way to protect my hair, and I love this leopard-skin print

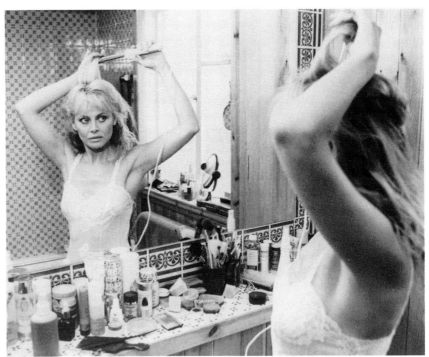

your hair down towards the ground, then dry with a blowdryer. By drying it against the way it falls, you put bounce into it. Then I simply part it in the middle, and that's it. Recently, though, I've had the crown slightly layered, giving me a sort of Bardot-ish look. While it is still damp I sweep the sides up into slides and let it dry thoroughly in that position. Later, when I take the slides out, it has dried with a bit of natural curve.

Every three or four months I drag out my set of heated rollers and I am always surprised that I don't remember from the last time that the result is a big let-down.

If I am playing a part that requires a set, big old-fashioned rollers work 100 per cent better. I partly dry my hair first to cut down on the time I need to spend under the dryer. I spray the whole lot with a little setting lotion, then roll it up. But I would never bother to do it unless I was being paid.

If you've got thick, curly hair, however, you might want to try setting it on huge rollers for a change to achieve a smooth look. But make sure it's bone dry before you take out the rollers. Use heated rollers and hair tongs only as a last resort if you've got a sudden invitation from the man of your dreams.

Coping with Fine Hair

This comes from the heart. Avoid an all-over layer cut, which I have found makes my hair look too thin. Fine hair does tend to look better a bit shorter, but only if you are slim enough to take it. Otherwise I'd just let it grow and to hell with the fact that it looks a bit straggly.

Hair thickeners do work but they tend to take the shine off your hair, so I just use them on the back, underneath hair. When your hair is wet, bend forwards and apply the thickener. I use Hair Thickener. Dry your hair in that position too, with a blowdryer, and you will find that the underneath hair dries with much more volume.

Invest in a diffuser attachment for your hairdryer, which looks like a shower head. If you've got curly or permed hair it is very effective, because it spreads the hot air to give a natural look, and it can really revive an old perm. Professional hairdressers use them, so ask yours if he can get one for you or try a good chemist's.

Another trick with fine hair is to have the underneath hair body permed. I'm not big on perms as a rule, but I have found that this method helps to make my hair look thicker and achieve that kind of pre-Raphaelite look which I can also get by using my soft rollers called Molton Browners.

Being on the move, it's important for me to establish relationships with hairdressers in each city where I spend time. I go to Benjamin in New York City, John Frieda in London and Michaeljohn in Los Angeles.

They introduced me to their Michaeljohn Mousse way back when I had short hair and wanted it to have that stand-up look. Today there are several mousses on the market, including one by L'Oréal. You use them on wet hair, then comb it into place. They're lighter than a regular setting lotion, but they do help a style stay put.

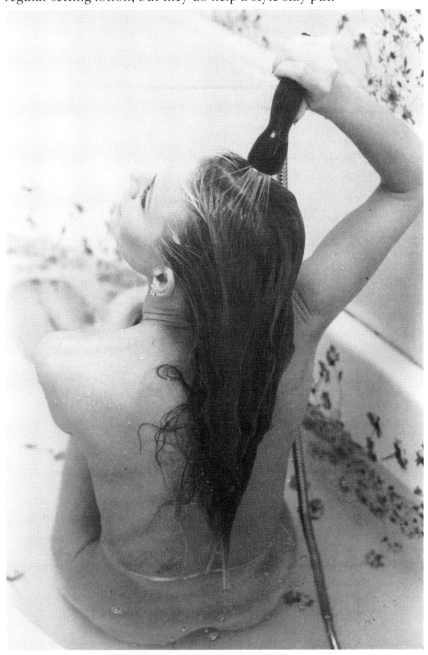

If you can bear it, a final cold rinse makes your hair shine

Following page: Two ways with the Heidi look – either plaited (top) or twisted (bottom)

39

Coping with Thick Hair

If you've got naturally thick, curly hair then keep it. If it's well cut it looks terrific. If it's too heavy around your face and tends to sit like a big woolly hat from ear to ear, ask your hairdresser to thin it out a bit. You can also try using combs and braids and twists to keep it away from your face. Or try putting half your hair up and leaving the rest down, so that it looks less weighty.

In Praise of Highlights

If you want to lighten the look of your hair, highlights are an infinitely more convenient method than bleaching and tinting. For instance, if you have dark hair and want to go blonde, or even just a few shades lighter, first the hairdresser has got to strip every ounce of colour out of your hair, which is a nightmare to do, then they have to put dye on top of that. Even if you stick close to your own colour, with an all-over permanent tint you have to tackle the regrowth in front every couple of weeks and the whole head every three or four weeks. It's a big commitment.

Highlights, on the other hand, take a long time to put in initially, but once they are in the upkeep is much easier. The fewer highlights you have, the less noticeable the regrowth, but they don't grow out in a hard line and you can always get away with a month between touch-ups.

I've managed to cope with highlights even on location in the far reaches of Thailand. You can always take your own bleach with you and brief a hairdresser to follow the existing pattern.

The finer the highlights, the more natural they look. You can put in masses to really lighten dark hair or you can go the other way and just have a half-inch strip around your face streaked.

My highlights stop smack on the crown of my head and round behind my ears, so that all my back and underneath hair is left its natural colour. Usually the underneath hair hasn't been tampered with or exposed to the light, and the colour can be very pretty. To me the darker hair underneath gives a more natural look when it peeps through than if I had a pure snow-white mat. Solid colour always looks more like a wig, more fake. It's most flattering to have your hair lighter up round your cheeks and eyes and a little darker down round the neck.

I tend to have more golden highlights because the camera likes them – ashy tones are too dull. But in life, ashy tones work well providing they don't get too grey. Ash blonde is what you want.

I recommend asking your hairdresser for two-tone streaks – alternate rows of ash and gold. If you have dark mouse or medium brown hair and you put in a whole batch of silvery streaks they will be very, very noticeable and your eye will easily be able to pick out the streaks. A mixture of colours blends better, looks much more natural and, if it's cleverly done, could pass for what you were born with.

If your hair is going grey, highlights are an excellent way to blend in the colour without anyone being any the wiser. If your hair is dark, chestnut or reddish gold highlights can lift it and give it life.

Whatever colour you are contemplating, the most important thing to consider is your skin tone. If you've got an olive-toned skin you are lucky and can get away with almost anything. But if you are dark with

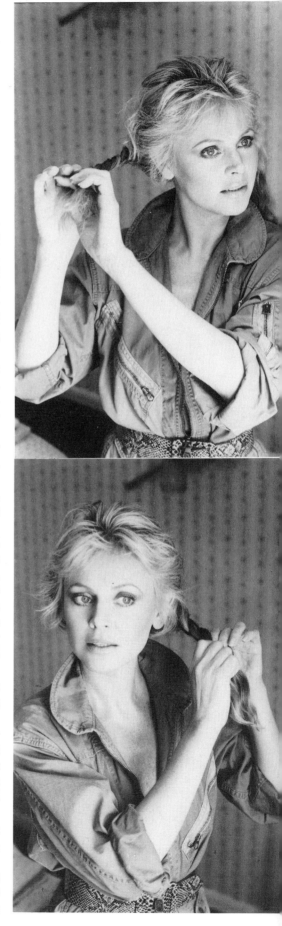

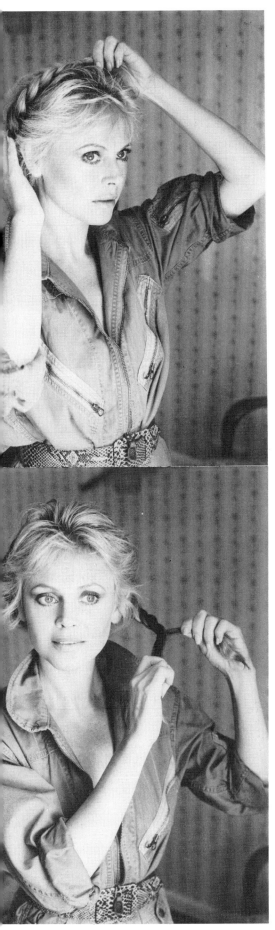

that translucent skin that has a tendency to look almost bluish, yellow and gold tones will be very unflattering and you are better off sticking to cool ash and beige tones.

Colourless henna has marvellous conditioning properties, but I wouldn't recommend red henna unless you are a redhead or have naturally dark hair. In about 1976 I was tired of being a streaky blonde and the idea of being a redhead suddenly appealed to me. Knowing that henna wasn't as damaging as tint, I went ahead. The result was disastrous. I didn't realize that the red henna would turn dark red on the virgin hair and light red on the streaks. My head resembled a red wool carpet. Soon after, I was offered a part in a film and the producers said, 'Of course for this role you'll be your natural blonde again.' I laughed and said, 'Of course!' I didn't realize that henna penetrates right through the hair shaft, so bleaching is virtually impossible.

If you're going to henna your hair red, unless it's very dark indeed snip a piece from under the back and test the colour before you go all the way. That goes for any hair colour you are contemplating. Forget about those peculiar hairdressers' lights that they claim are daylight – very untrustworthy. And forget about those dreadful little sample colour swatches. Insist on seeing the colour in daylight before you make up your mind.

One last word of warning about highlights – all good hairdressers use aluminium foil these days. If you spot a swimming cap and crochet hook, run a mile!

Putting It Up

Keep it simple. Rather than contorting your hair into the traditional confines of the french pleat, try this. Bend over, brush all your hair forward and just grab it into a bunch at the edge of your forehead. Catch it in an elastic band, stand up and twirl the hair round into a little knot. Don't worry about the back bits falling loose – that just gives you a softer, prettier profile. If that doesn't happen naturally, you can take a comb or use your fingers to pull a couple of little tendrils around your face. Don't pull the bun too tight, whatever you do. Most women look better with a softer line, and in my case it has the added advantage of hiding my ears. You can build up the knot with false pieces or decorate it with pins or combs. You can even put a stocking into a silk scarf and then tie it around the knot to give it more bulk.

It's fun to play with your hair and I am always experimenting. I have just rediscovered the old fifties' half-ponytail look. You section off the hair just above and behind your ears and fix it into a ponytail and just let the rest hang down. You can put a ribbon round the ponytail, or plait it, or even add a false piece.

The Heidi look also looks good. Just part your hair down the centre and section off enough hair above each ear to make into braids. Plait the hair on each side, then bring the braids up to the top of your head and pin into place.

As an alternative to plaiting, divide each side into two sections instead of three, and twirl the two sections round and round each other. Do this while your hair is still damp, or else dampen it. Put a heavy clip at the end of each twirl to keep it in position until the hair is dry. Pin up. The twists look very pretty.

When you put your hair up, don't do a beautiful job and then forget that there are forty-five pins visible to the world at the back. Mirrors aren't narcissistic – they make sense.

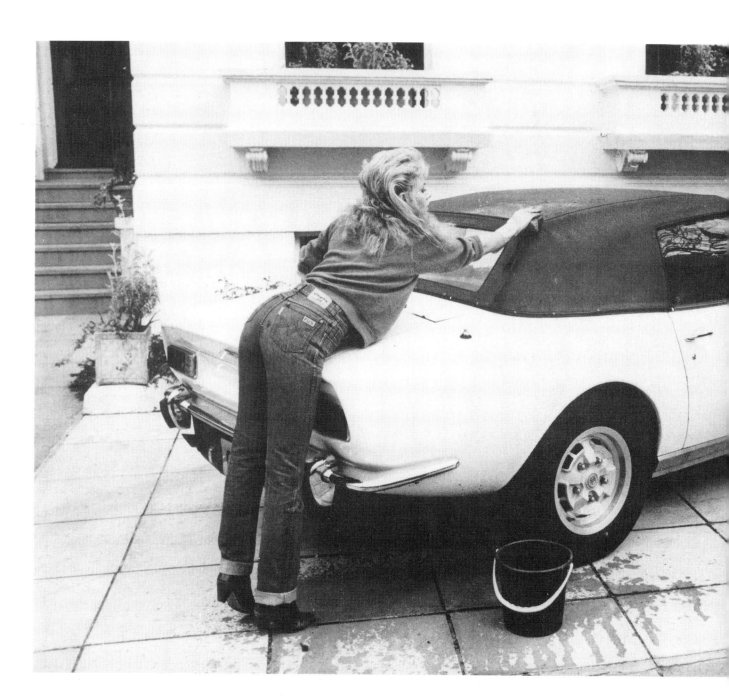

5/NAILS: GETTING THE RIGHT TOUCH

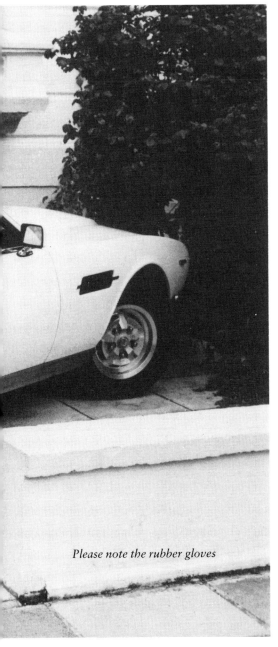

Please note the rubber gloves

Remember that old saying, 'You can never be too thin or too rich'? I'm adding, 'Your nails can never be too long.' Men like long nails. In those old forties' movies, couples were always scratching each other's backs, moaning and groaning. Claw marks down the back were the sure sign that sex had taken place.

In *Funny Girl*, Barbara Streisand's nails were incredibly long and I for one looked at nothing else. Those nails were almost obscene. That's why I would never wear red polish in a film. Who wants to be upstaged by a set of red talons?

I always dress in red for the Christmas Day festivities and break away from my neutral nail polish shade and wear red to match – but only if my nails are long enough to carry it off. There's nothing more horrible than short, stubby nails painted bright red. Hands and nails are very important but very neglected. Most people think the occasional scrub is sufficient, and it would never cross their minds even to use hand cream.

Nails can be a great asset but you really have to love them, otherwise there is no point in having them because they can be a terrible nuisance. Nails are a far more serious business in the States. No one laughs at someone opening a car door with their elbow or pushing lift buttons with a knuckle. It goes without saying they're protecting their nails.

My nails are the real thing, never touched by anything false. And for those sceptics who imagine they are the result of unfamiliarity with housework, I've got news for you! I collect silver and one of my passions in life is polishing it. I occasionally scrub my kitchen floor. I can and do polish my furniture. I paint and I don't mean pictures. I do front door steps, window frames, the lot. I do all my own gardening and I even wash my own car. But I *do* take good care of my nails.

Rubber gloves are cumbersome but what you can do – I know it sounds obscene – is use close-fitting surgical gloves. They're ideal for fiddly tasks like silver cleaning. When I wash the car or the windows I wear little cotton gloves, then rubber gloves on top – somehow the cotton gloves make the rubber ones more manageable. I garden in woolly knitted gloves topped with rubber gloves. In cold weather I won't go anywhere without a pair of gloves.

I recommend that everyone has a professional manicure – I sent Victoria for her first when she was thirteen. Concentrate on what the manicurist is doing and try to memorize her method so that you can copy it at home. When I'm in Los Angeles I have a manicure once a week. In England I do it myself – unfortunately I don't find English manicurists as skilful in dealing with my American nail shape.

If you grew up in Europe, like me, you probably had short, stubby nails because you either bit them or were instructed to cut them that way. Peering at our elders, we were confronted with these sharp, pointed weapons that ruined stockings and underwear. We were looking at the 'perfect nail' – the one you could kill with. But that did not mean the good, strong nail, because filing the sides down to the quick and filing the top to a point weakened them very badly.

I never had a set of nails to speak of until I reached California and found there was another kind of nail. Today I wouldn't dream of filing down the sides: I file them straight across and they are incredibly strong. If you still have the old pointed shape, sorry, but you have to cut the points off and start afresh, it's the only way. Keep them dead straight across and only shape them when they're really long and then just at the point.

On average nails grow one and a half inches a year. They're made of keratin which is also found in skin and hair. People ask me why my nails grow so fast? I truly believe it is the vitamin-mineral compounds that make nails grow long and strong (and hair too for that matter), so take a high-potency multi-vitamin with minerals in it.

Tips for Tired Nails

Olive Oil Treat

I remember my mother heating a small bowl of olive oil over a pan of water until the oil was warm. Then she would sit with her fingers dipped in the oil for about fifteen minutes. Like a lot of old-fashioned remedies, it works well, softening and nourishing the skin and cuticles. I do this every three months or so.

Overnight Pack

You could inform your man that you're going to bed with your gloves on, but it's probably best kept for nights when you sleep alone. This pack is really gooey but terrifically softening. I put big globs of hand lotion, olive oil and almond oil on my hands, plus a lavish helping of cuticle cream on my nails, working it in well.

Over that lot I put thick white cotton utility gloves from Woolworth's. I promise you that in the morning your hands will look and feel fabulous.

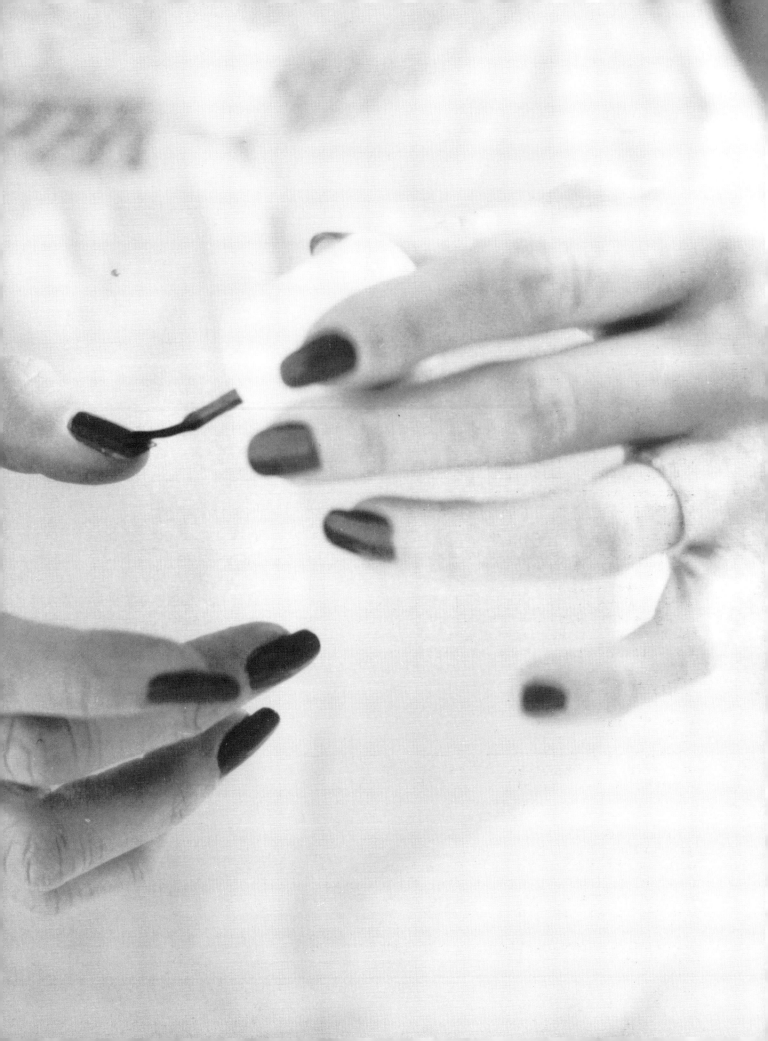

Flying's Drying
Never take off without a small pot of rich hand cream or moisturizing cream in your travel kit.

Quick Cuticle Trick
Push back your cuticles with the towel whenever you wash your hands. It's an old-fashioned remedy again, but it works if you do it regularly.

Home Manicure Routine

I know you've been saving your nails for the last two years and the thought of taking scissors to them fills you with horror, but if you've got pointed talons – I call them little boats – my advice is to cut them right off.

Usually women with little boats tend to have one short boat, two medium boats and a whole collection of different lengths on display. It's vital to keep your nails the same length, whatever that length may be. If one has broken off short, bring the others into line. That, I promise, is the most painful part, so grit your teeth and read on.

At Night
1. Remove all the old polish with good old-fashioned Cutex. It's not on your nails long enough to dry them out, and oily remover is too sticky.

2. Cut them dead straight across as if you're cutting a sheet of paper.

3. File with an emery board, rough side first, not to round them but just to get the sharp bits smoothed off. File from sides to centre, and don't saw back and forth. Angle the board so it is filing the back rather than the front of the nail edge. Never use a metal file, which tears at the delicate keratin layers.

4. If you've been wearing red varnish without undercoat or basecoat, your nails are no doubt stained reddish brown. The only way to shift that is to soak them in peroxide or bleach for a couple of minutes, but be very careful – if you've got any little tears in the cuticles you will scream.
If that doesn't work, take the soft side of an emery board and gently file the entire surface of each clean nail.

5. Give your nails a good scrub with a nailbrush. Push the cuticles back as you go.

Next Day
Don't start two minutes before you are due to leave the house or put on your stockings. Basecoat and ridge filler take about sixty seconds each to dry, while polish takes considerably longer.

1. If you've got a tear in your tenth nail and the other nine are perfect, fix it with a nail repair kit. L'Oréal, Max Factor and Revlon make them and they come complete with instructions. Before you start, make sure the nail is scrupulously clean with no residue of soap or grease on it. File over the tear very carefully on the top surface of the nail so that it's roughened a little, which I've found makes the glue hold better. For anything trickier than a small tear, I'd go to a professional every time.

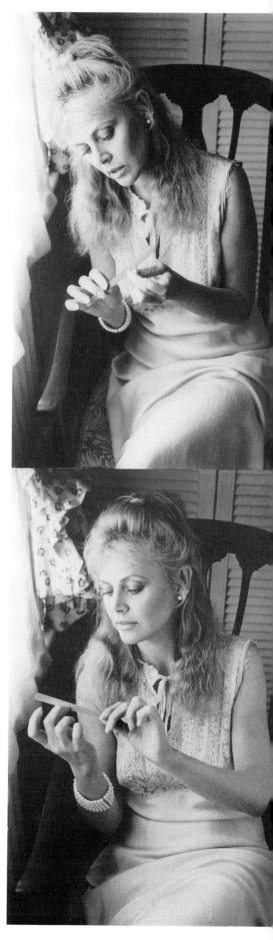

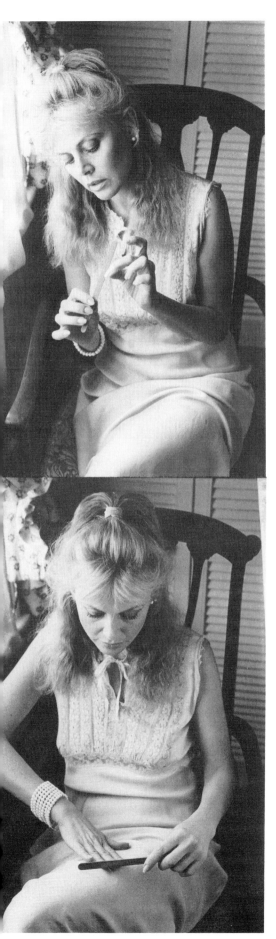

2. Check your nails for ridges (see 3). Take an undercoat or basecoat and paint it on your nails, brushing under the tips too. Don't put too much on the brush or it will smear. Keep an orange stick handy to clean up mistakes. The best way is to brush most of the polish off inside the bottle and work with a fairly dry brush.

Basecoat should be very thin. It's just there to protect your natural nail colour by putting a barrier between it and the polish. I find the best method is to make the first brush stroke from cuticle to tip, in the centre of the nail, then to fill in with strokes each side.

3. Look at your nails from all angles. Do they resemble railway tracks? Ridges are often a sign of poor health – or simply old age – but vitamin A, iodine, and calcium can help. Ridges show up even more with polish, so either gently file down the entire surface of your nails with the soft side of an emery board before using basecoat, or, alternatively, use a ridge filler after your basecoat. Chanel make a particularly good one which fills in all those little railway tracks.

4. If you have time, apply a second basecoat, but it's not essential. What is essential is to let each coat dry thoroughly before applying the next.

5. Put on two coats of polish, then follow with a fast-drying top coat. For some reason they're oil-based but they do work well. Wait at least thirty seconds after painting your nails before using the fast dry, and then sit tight for a minimum of ten minutes. If you've done a good job and the polish looks really pretty, there is nothing more destructive than a smudge. I'm the most impatient person in the world but it's worth waiting.

6. The only maintenance needed is to add another layer of colour or top coat every other day, just to keep your nails in tip-top condition.

The Colour Debate

When I was eighteen, someone informed me that pearl nail polish was worn only by au pair girls, 'Foreign, of course', and for that reason you will never see me wearing it. Some things just stick. To my mind a pearlized nail looks common. I know all nail polish manufacturers are going to kill me but pearly orange, white or pink of any kind do not cross my dressing table. Red pearls are the only exception. Pearls have a very fifties' look and go hand in hand with chalky lips and stiff petticoats.

On a more rational note, I also give all the crazy nail colours a wide berth – mainly, I admit, since I find them a distraction, particularly on the screen.

Unless you have extremely well-manicured nails, don't wear colour except for a special party. If you're going to wear a red dress, red stockings and a red rose in your hair, why not wear red nails? But don't then keep them for the next three days, clashing horribly with your everyday wardrobe. If you wear red you've got to be prepared to take it off once it has served its purpose.

I would never go out wearing a red dress with burgundy nails. If I couldn't be bothered to change my polish I would change my dress. It's very unpleasant to have clashing colours if the nails are prominent.

I would also stay away from the whole brown scale, including all those autumn rusts. At one time dark brown talons were the trademark of people like Diana Ross and Cher, but those colours have been done to death now. In a cold climate it's wise to stay away from anything with blue tones in it, which includes all those mauvey pinks and shocking pink. They just don't look good with blue flesh.

I don't think anyone needs to own more than three shades nowadays: very pale pink, dark beige, and red. Day-to-day dark beige with a hint of pink in it will go with everything from evening gowns to jeans and sweatsuits. I wear my beige colour to exercise class or to a ball, with or without jewellery. From these three basic shades you can concoct pretty much every colour you are likely to need. I keep a spare empty bottle and, since all polish ingredients are basically the same, just blend up the shade I need.

If you are wearing jewellery, decide what you want to emphasize – your nails or your diamonds. If you've got burgundy red nails and a beautiful cluster of rubies or emeralds, the polish can really detract from the jewellery. Unless you can find an exact match to the stone, it's safer to stick with a neutral beige polish and let your jewellery have centre stage. Rubies, for instance, tend to be a little more blue in tone than orange, and if you wear an orangey red it will kill the colour of the stone.

Grandma's White Moon Trick

My grandmother used to paint her nails with a pale, transparent polish leaving the half moons white. It's fiddly to do yourself so I ask the manicurist to do it for me. She paints the half moons in with a white polish and also paints the tips of the nails white. It looks very effective.

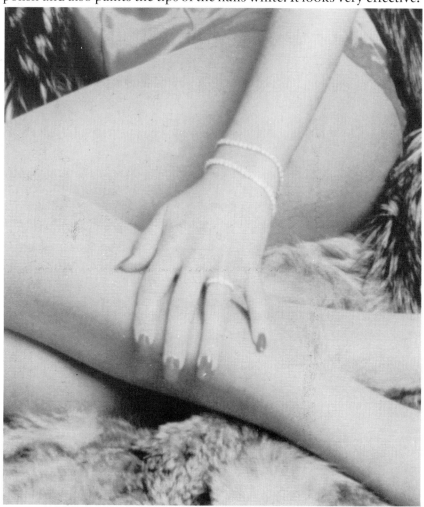

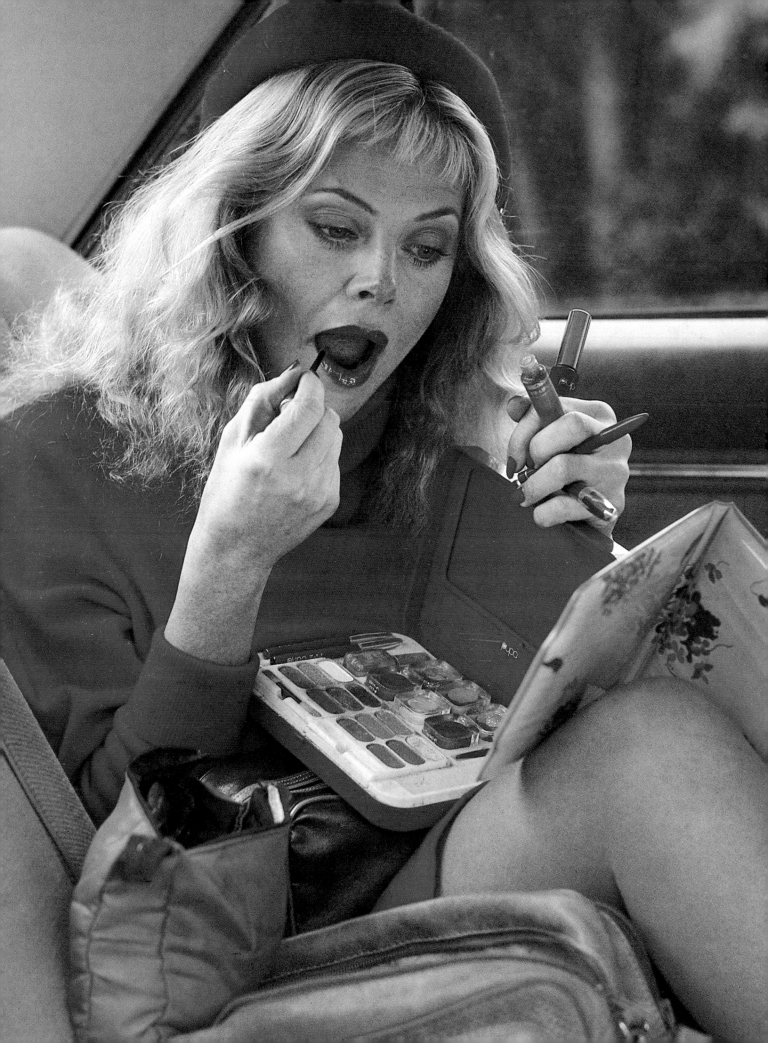

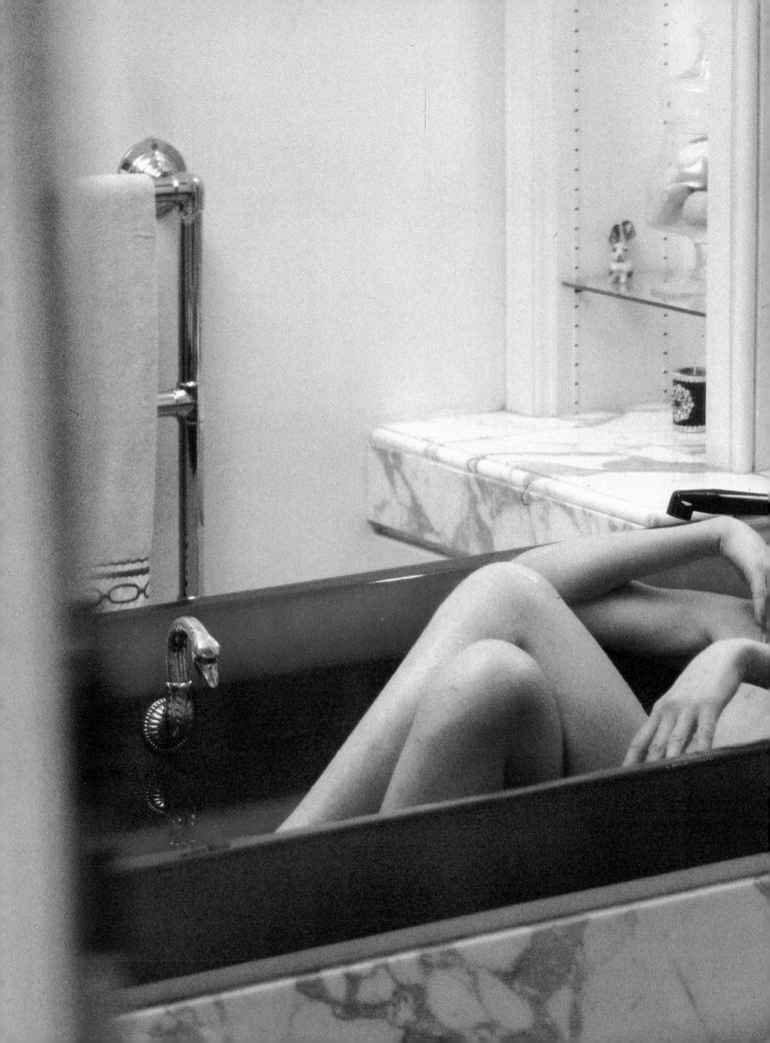

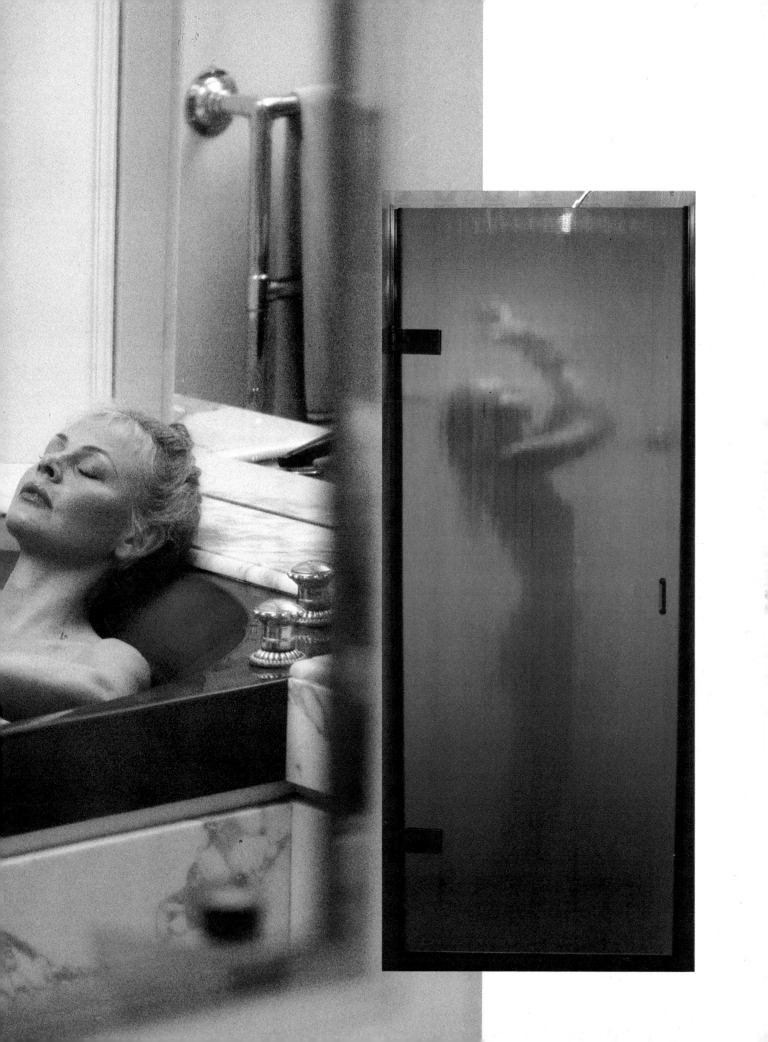

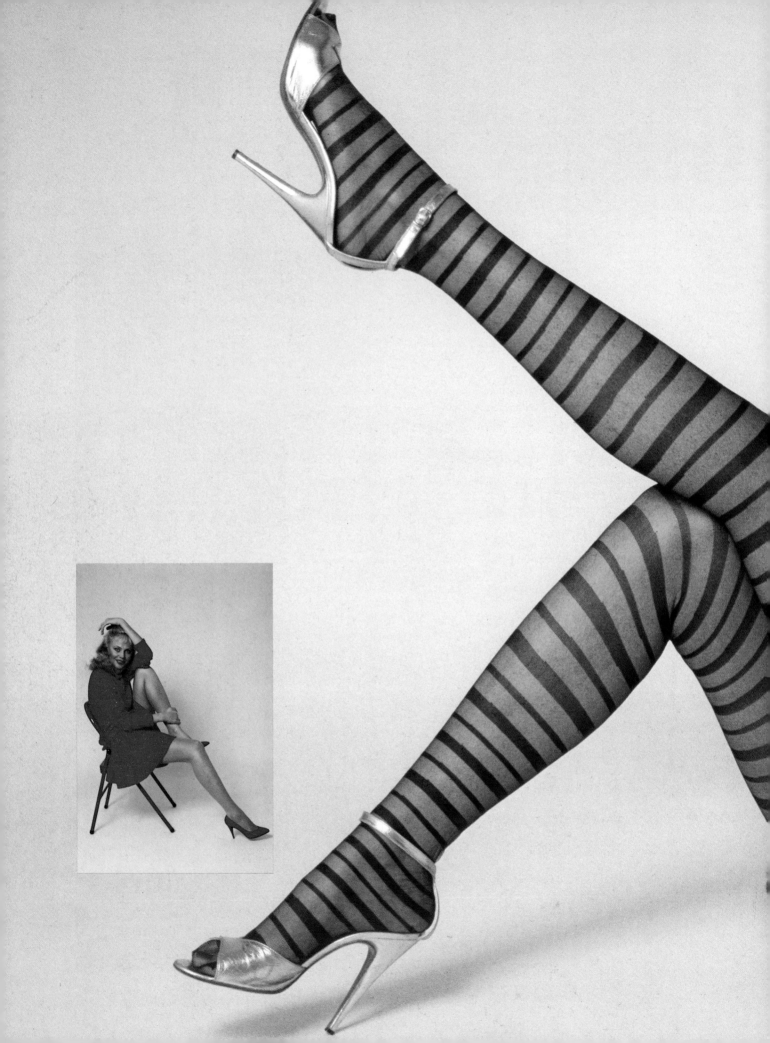

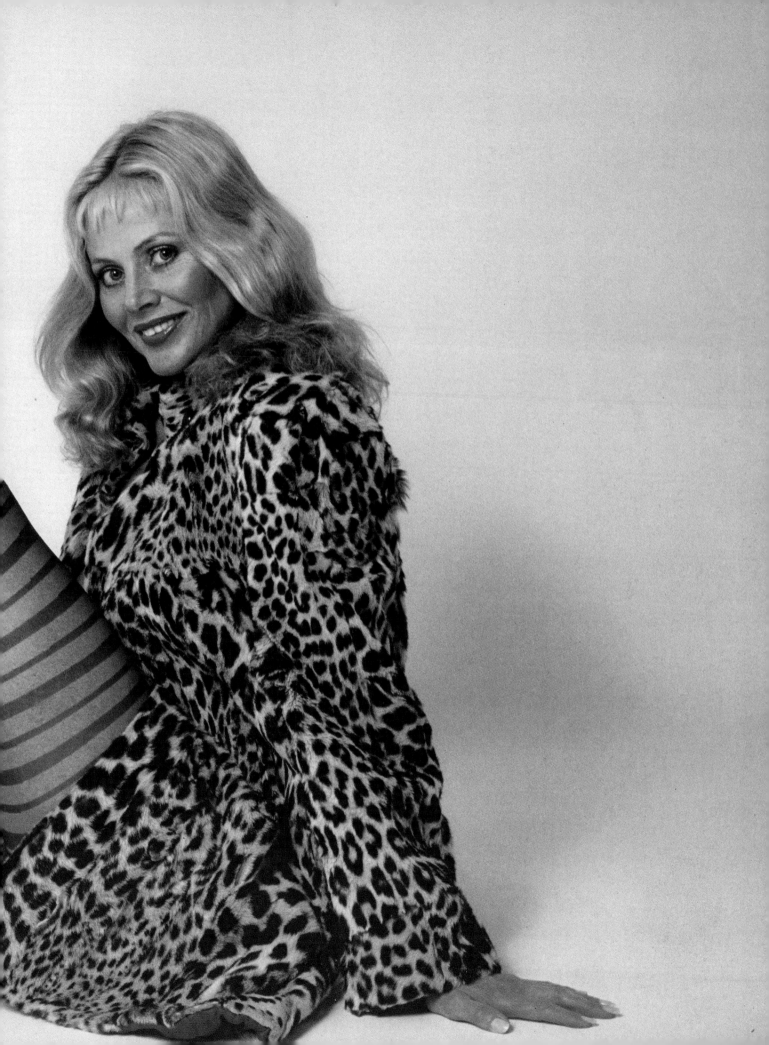

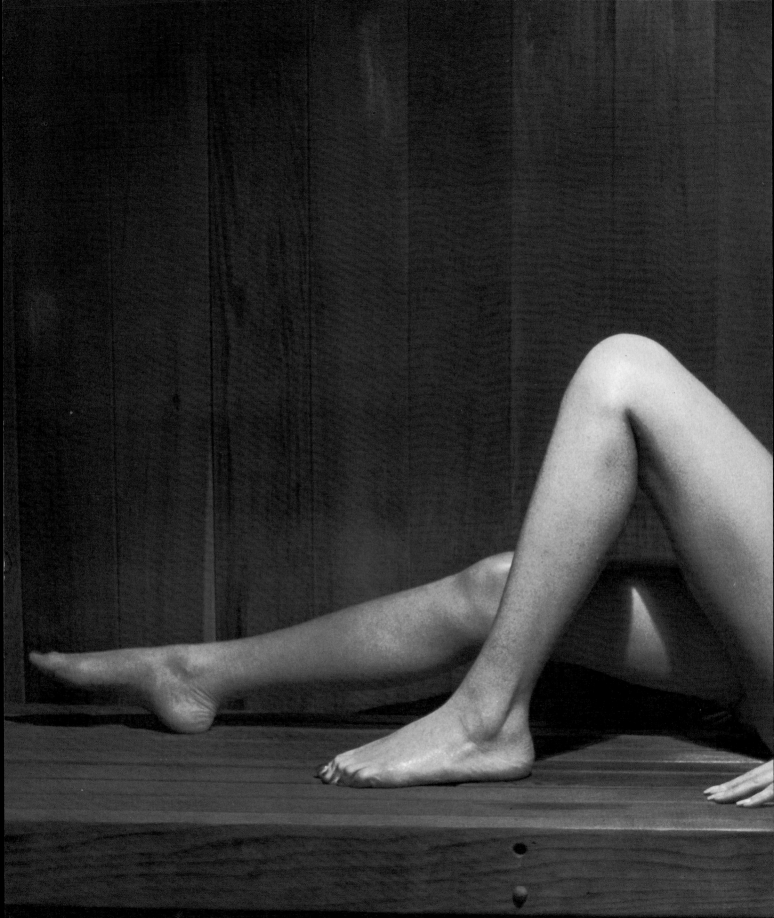

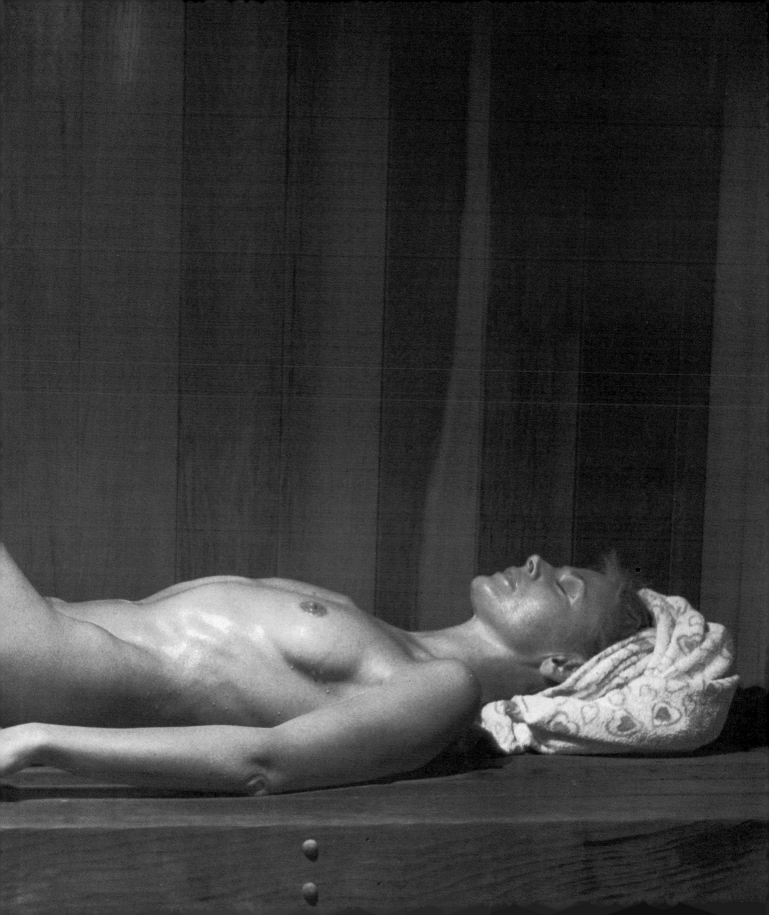

6 / TEETH: SOMETHING TO SMILE ABOUT

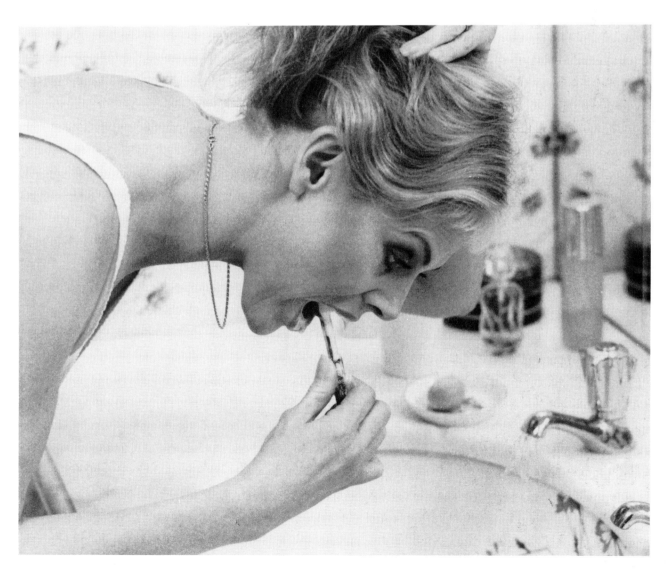

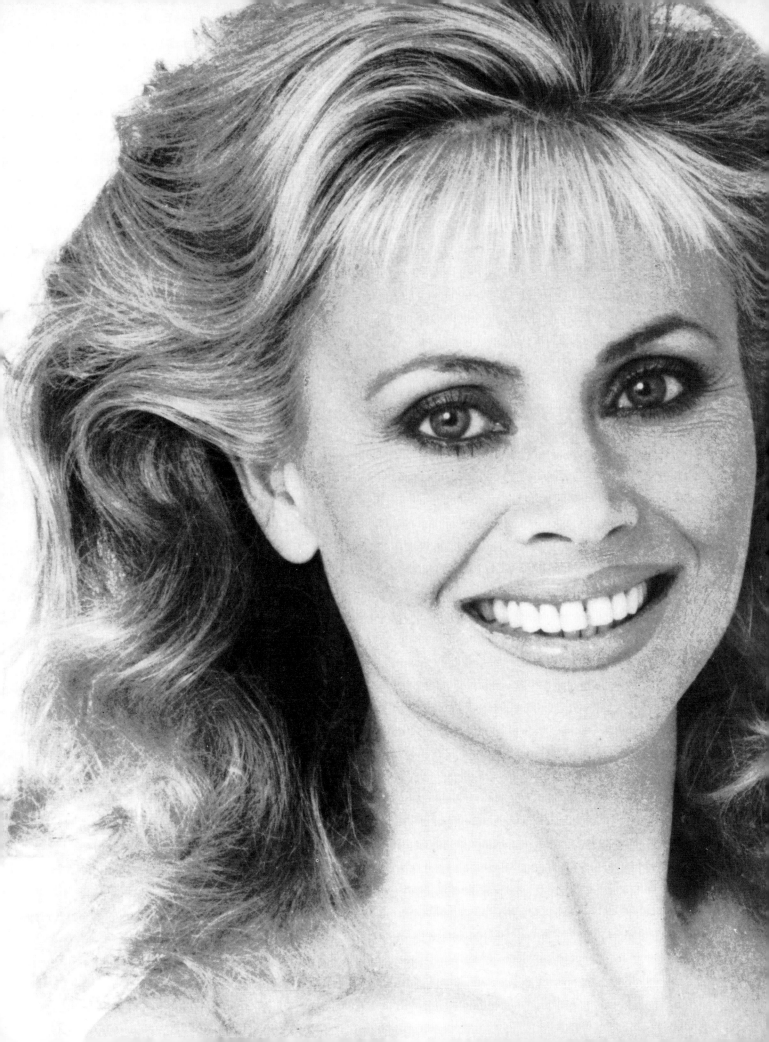

Few things are more off-putting than a grotty mouth, and I know men feel just as strongly about that. They will sit and drool all night over a gorgeous blonde, unable to understand why she's alone and hasn't disappeared with someone. Invariably it's because when she opens her mouth she sends everyone running.

War babies generally have bad teeth and I am no exception. Despite my parents telling me that sugar was bad for me, I ate so many sweeties that I had more cavities than you can imagine. They told me to brush my teeth thoroughly twice a day, but unfortunately I showed singular disregard for such sound advice. The free school dentistry in my day followed the philosophy of, 'Drill a hole, fill it with silver and send 'em home.'

Now capping is to me something akin to plastic surgery. It's heaven. I wouldn't take perfectly healthy teeth and cap them, obviously, but all those childhood fillings eventually crumble away and when they do it's time to invest in caps if you can possibly afford them. I finally fulfilled my dream when I was thirty-five. I'm not ashamed to say that I had every single tooth capped with the exception of my front teeth and four at the bottom – they didn't need it. I would always choose that as the first investment to make in your body. Get your mouth in order, then have your eyes fixed, your breasts lifted or whatever else you choose.

Obviously smoking doesn't help the state of your teeth, but that's a personal decision. Smokers' toothpastes are reasonably efficient at removing the yellow stains in the front, but a cleaning session with the dentist is best.

Fortunately today there is far more emphasis on preventive dentistry – how to keep them rather than how to mend them. Hair and nails will grow again, but if you abuse your teeth you are going to be stuck with the result for a very long time. Flossing can save you an awful lot of dental trouble if you start early enough. I've flossed my teeth since I had them capped, because it helps prevent gum infection. I have a dental check-up and professional cleaning every six months and cannot recommend highly enough that you do the same. At the slightest twinge of pain I see my dentist. Whatever fears you may have, believe me, it's better to go immediately than to put it off and end up needing a root canal.

If your gums bleed when you clean your teeth you could well be suffering from a vitamin deficiency, but it could be an infection so don't hesitate to get professional advice.

Most people brush their teeth regularly but incorrectly. If you brush them from side to side you'll remove all the natural enamel. You should brush down over your top teeth and up over the bottom ones, including your gums in the brush strokes.

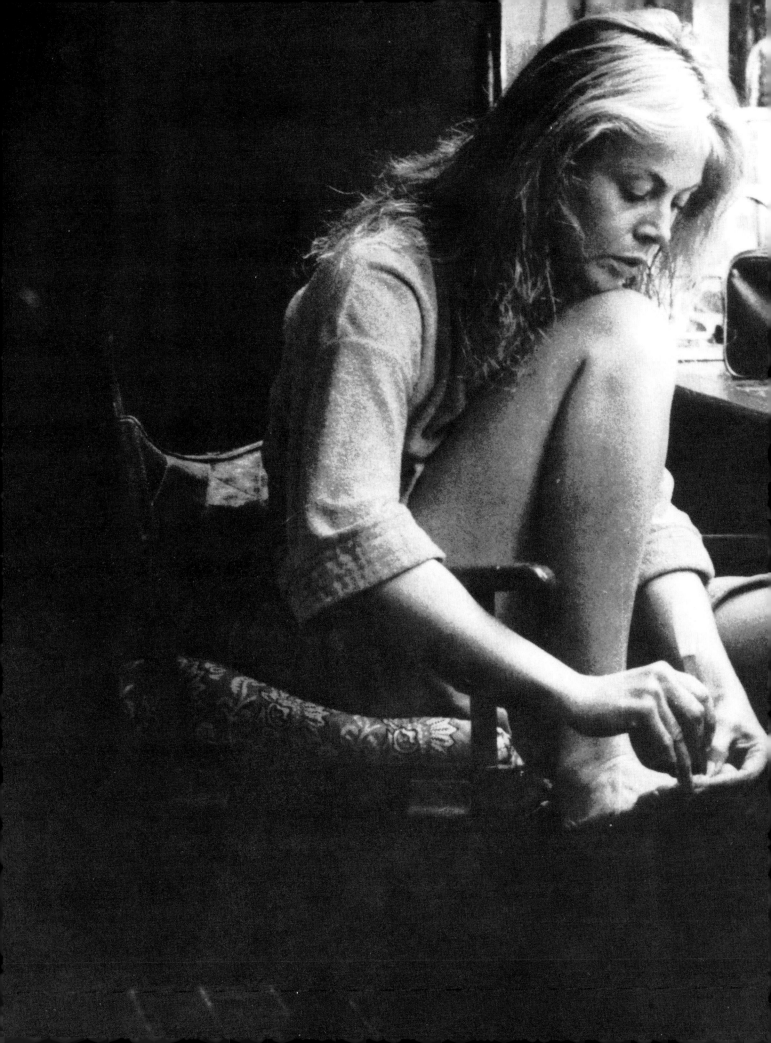

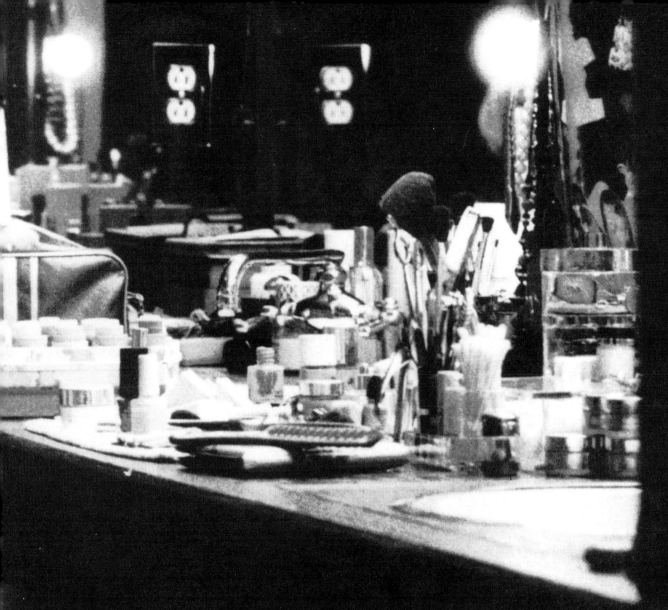

7 / THE WORLD AT YOUR FEET

I believe a good-looking foot is as important as a good-looking hand.
I'm not saying there is necessarily anything very sensual about feet, but
after all they have been known to touch a man's lips, and obviously in
the dark the poor soul isn't going to know what he's reaching for, so
it's really up to you! If that's the kind of intimate relationship you
have, you have to keep your feet lovable.

To most of us, feet are nothing more than objects you stick shoes on.
If we were lucky our mothers sensibly forced us into highly unsexy
walking boats when our feet were still at the formative stage. Of course
there is no telling how much harm we did as teenagers by forcing our

way into shoes a half-size too small. I vividly remember evenings of sheer hell rammed into unnaturally pointed shoes, and the legacy of that was corns at best, malformation at worst.

One advantage of growing up in the Swedish countryside was that, thanks to the climate, the times when we could wear high heels were few and far between. Consequently my feet were relatively good until I moved to Los Angeles and got into Frederick's of Hollywood's '**** me' shoes, which are as high as hell and pointed and literally only fit for walking from one side of the bed to the other.

Simple Foot Care

Like a manicure, a pedicure is a really good investment. Visit a chiropodist first if your feet are in disgusting shape or they hurt you.

Examine your feet at as close quarters as your dexterity will allow. Run your hand over the soles after a bath and you may well find that your little toes have formed their own mountain wedge that you could almost cut a cake with, and that your heel is fit to sandpaper a wall. In case you didn't know it, a chiropodist can whisk off that whole dead top layer and leave you feeling like a new woman.

The alternative is to work on the hard skin yourself. I always wondered what my mother did with that peculiar grey object, the pumice stone. Now I know. These days there are gadgets that look like metallic pot scourers and they work well too.

I try to give myself a simple pedicure at least once a month.

1. Remove all old nail varnish so that the sins that lurk behind the big toenail will be revealed. Use the same method as for a manicure.

2. If you wear tights or stockings, it's much kinder on them if you cut your nails straight across and file them smooth with an emery board.

3. You can give your feet some tough treatment by cleaning them with a good, hard scrub with a nailbrush. Don't be afraid of putting an implement behind the nail and removing half of last year's garden, last summer's beach or whatever else is lurking there.

4. If your toenails are ridged, plane the surface down with the smooth side of an emery board.

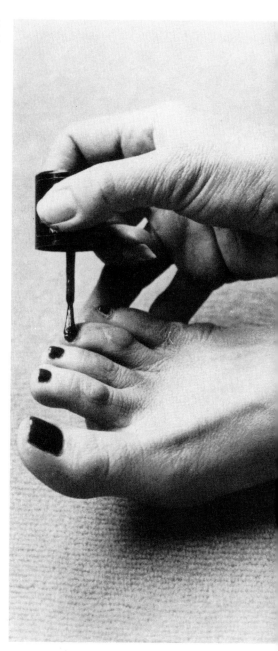

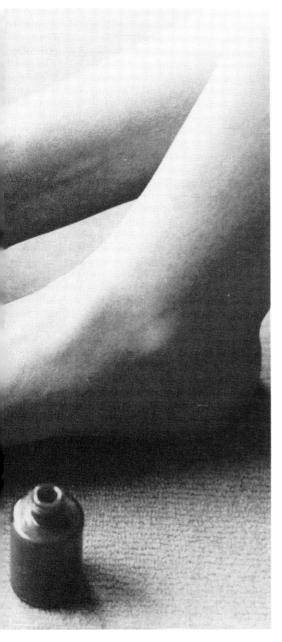

5. Cuticle remover works even better on toenails, for some reason, so if your cuticles have crept halfway up your nails and are ugly and straggly, smooth cuticle remover right around the edges of your nails, then scrub off briskly when it's had time to work.

6. When you put body lotion on your legs, remember to include the soles of your feet and around your heels. They're especially prone to dry skin and this is a long-term policy that can make the world of difference. If they are very rough, try using cuticle remover there too. I hate to think what it would do to wood or china, but it certainly softens hard skin.

Whenever I put lotion on my legs or feet I make a point of standing with my legs dead straight and bending from the waist. I make it a daily routine. Most people have a big of saggy, bulging flesh on the backs of their thighs below the bum because it never gets a stretch.

7. Most women have the odd hair or two growing on their toes, and frankly it's not very sensual. Snip them off before they grow into a little forest.

8. If you want to use polish I suggest basecoat followed by clear topcoat, although red's a glamorous alternative if you're wearing sexy open-toed sandals. For everyday I prefer to keep my toenails natural but shiny, and buffing really makes them look good. Buy an old-fashioned buffer and just go hell for leather across your nails. Once a month should do the trick.

Foot Treat

Some beauty salons have electric mittens and bootees that they put on over an oil pack. It's almost like wearing a hot blanket and it makes your skin more receptive to the oil. Sometimes I indulge in a treatment, or you can copy the idea at home.

Put almond oil on your feet. Rub it in well, then put a plastic bag over each foot. Top that off with a pair of old socks and go to bed.

Be careful when you step into the shower the next morning because you will slip all over the place. You can forget the plastic bags if you wish, but they do keep the oil from soaking into your socks.

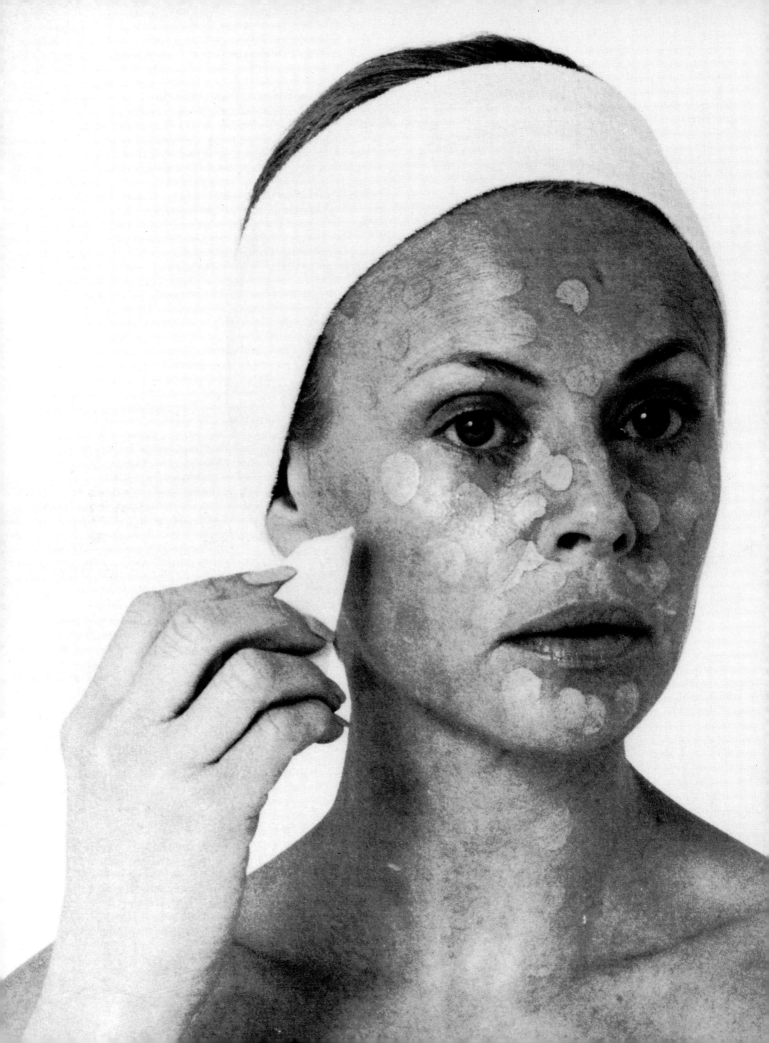

8/MAKING FACES

I'm a woman and I'm vain and I really don't want anyone to see me without make-up in public. I don't feel I have to put on a pretty face for a man, although usually one does to start with. But if he say he loves you the way you are, you take his word for it and you live happily ever after until you find someone else!

I believe in make-up and I'm living proof that it won't destroy your skin and that mascara won't make all your eyelashes fall out. I don't want to give the impression that I'm caked in make-up by the time I'm finished – far from it. But there is a whole art in making up to look as though you're not really made up. It takes time, and don't believe a word of it when you read that models hop out of bed, pull on their jeans, dab on a bit of blusher and instantly look gorgeous. That's rubbish. That's not what they do. They put the full works on and it *looks* as though they're just wearing a bit of blusher and mascara because they're good at using make-up. No one, unless they're eighteen and tanned, can just hop out of bed and look terrific. So the secret is to use make-up skilfully to achieve what I call a slightly overdone, natural look.

Here's my basic routine, which is second nature to me now and impervious to passing trends. It sounds complicated but in fact each step takes no time at all, especially when you're used to it.

The Britt Make-up Routine

1. Moisturize your skin. No make-up will go on properly if your skin is dry and patchy.

2. Pale liquid make-up base comes next (**A**). I don't skimp on it – if you do, it streaks – and rub it in well with fingers or sponge, working up to the hairline, across the eyelids, and into the crevices around my nose. I stretch my mouth so it gets into all the little creases around my lips, and then when my face is smooth I start blending it down my neck right to the collarbone and right round behind my ears and down below them. Since it's unlikely that the colour matches your skin exactly, it's vital that you don't miss anything. Make absolutely sure that your make-up does not end in a stripe at the side of your face or chin, which can ruin an otherwise perfect make-up. It's not enough just to look straight into a mirror – you should always take a second mirror and check side views.

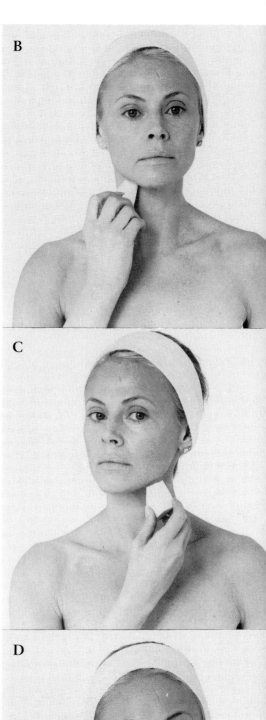

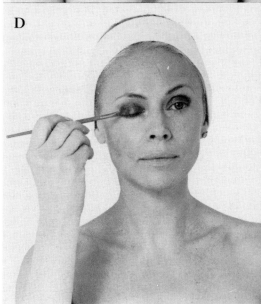

3. I take a dry, white, triangular cosmetic sponge (**B, C**) and remove any excess make-up. Why not put on less in the first place, you might wonder. Well, if you use too little it doesn't blend as evenly, and it's harder to add more than to sponge off any extra.

Make-up people throw away a sponge after every session, but I wash mine out and keep using it for a couple of weeks.

4. I take a light-coloured under-eye cover-up (my favourite is Erno Laszlo) and put it on to my fingertip. From there I pat it on under my eyes to blot out shadows and stroke it out at the sides towards the hairline.

If you use a stick, never put the make-up on straight from the stick because it drags the skin. Putting it on your finger warms it up and makes it easier to apply.

If you're not exactly sure where to put it, *tilt* your head down and look in the mirror so you get a clearer view of the hollow dark circles under your eyes that you're looking for.

5. I take a white pencil (Lyla hypo-allergenic) and draw a white line around the edge of my mouth. Then I pout to locate those tiny wrinkles around my mouth and I draw a white line in each of them.

I also draw a white line on the two lines that run from nose to mouth and in the lines that go out from the sides of my nose. With my fingertip or cosmetic sponge I gently pat over the white lines to soften them.

6. Next I brush on a lightish brown shadow (**D, E**). Whether you're blonde, brunette or redhead, always steer clear of red tones when you're buying brown shadow. They bring out the red in your eyes and that's the last thing you want. Ash tones are more flattering. I brush it just above the lashes on the top lid right across the socket and out to the eyebrow, and right below the lower lashes.

Be careful not to use too much powder on the brush – it can fall on to your cheeks and ruin everything. If it should happen, put a little foundation on the sponge and gently rub until it's disappeared.

7. Next I powder the lot with loose, translucent powder and a big, fluffy brush (**F**). Marlene Dietrich said, 'Never powder under your eyes' and I follow her advice, because powder just shows up wrinkles. Just powder from the inner corner of your eye, though, to about the middle of your eye. Powder right across your forehead and all the way down the neck.

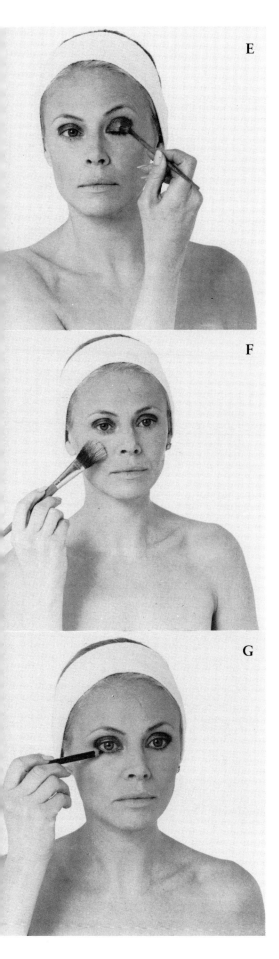

E

F

G

8. Let the whole lot set for a few minutes, then check to see if you've put too much powder or make-up anywhere. If you have, it's simple to sponge it off.

9. I keep a toothbrush handy to brush excess make-up and powder out of my eyebrows, then I pencil them with a mousey shade (Maybelline brown). In the past I have bleached my brows, not to mention plucked them out of existence, but now they've grown back to their natural colour. Blondes in particular have to watch out for pencils with any kind of ginger in them. That looks awful and is worse than going too dark. Dark brows, particularly if you were born with them, are to my mind very beautiful.

10. The next step is to stroke a little black shadow close to my eyelashes, just on the outer half of my eyes, halfway along the top lid and halfway along the bottom lid (**G**).

11. I take a white, pearlized shadow and put a little line in the middle of the upper eyelid very close to the lashes; then I stroke it on to the browbone up to the brow as a highlight (**H, I**).

12. I have a small pot of white, non-pearlized highlight powder, and I use that or a beigey-white powder and just brush between my eyebrows down around the inner eye corners and down over the lines from nose to mouth – it softens them.

13. I curl my eyelashes, three times for each eye (**J**)

14. I bite on a clean sponge to take all the make-up off my lips and immediately put on Elizabeth Arden's Eight Hour Cream which I keep by me at all times. Alternatively, if you intend to use lipstick you can powder over your lips without cleaning off the make-up. It provides a base that helps hold the lipstick colour.

15. I take a silvery-blue or grey, hypo-allergenic pencil (Lyla again) and I use that just round the inside edge of my lower lids (**K**).

16. Next I use powder blusher (**L**). As a general guideline, I believe the less red in the colour the better. I use a flat, fan-shaped brush to apply it.

The most common mistake women make – and I have to include myself in this – is to shade the whole lot right down to the jawline. Apart from looking artificial you also end up looking as though you've grown a beard.

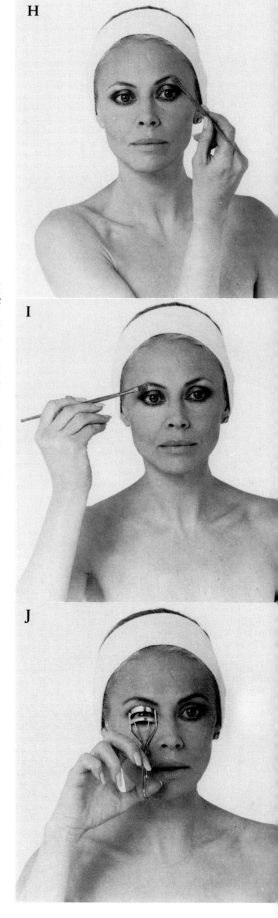

The best way is to suck in your cheeks as if your life depended on it. I don't care how chubby your face is, you are going to find some sort of bone line underneath and that's where the shading should go. Brush the blusher on from the edge of your face to the centre of your cheeks. Don't go one step further, or you'll have the Salvador Dali look.

Blend the blusher in but always use upward brush strokes. Don't take the colour any lower, otherwise you'll look as though you've got five o'clock shadow, but a touch at the temples is effective.

17. I have my eyelashes dyed blue-black which is wonderful for the summer and gives the look of mascara when you wake up in the morning and when you dip in the pool.

However, mascara makes a make-up come alive. In this day and age it's too boring to spit and rub with a cake mascara so I always use a roll-on, but without the little bits in it. I spend as long on my mascara as on the rest of my make-up put together.

First look down and mascara the tops of your top lashes, then look up and mascara underneath the top lashes. Next mascara the bottom lashes.

Clogged mascara looks terrible, so always separate the lashes with the mascara brush. I have a little lash comb that also does the trick very well.

When you use mascara you should always have a sponge ready to rescue any specks that fall on to your cheeks.

Incidentally, I have two tricks when I buy new mascara. First, I always curve the brush a little bit to match the shape of my eye, and leave it in the wand like that. Second, new mascara is awful to work with because it comes out in big, runny blobs. The older it gets, the better I like it. So when I buy a new one I pull the brush out and leave it out overnight in the bathroom to dry a bit before I start using it.

18. Lips come last, and a lot depends on climate. If you live in a cold place you are very restricted in the colours you can wear because almost all shades look dreadful with blue skin. In a warm climate, pretty much anything goes.

Personally I don't wear strong lip colours unless I'm going all out for glamour because my lips are very big. Particularly on the screen, great big red lips look like some kind of monstrosity approaching when you speak.

Having taken my white or skin-tone pencil around my lips at the

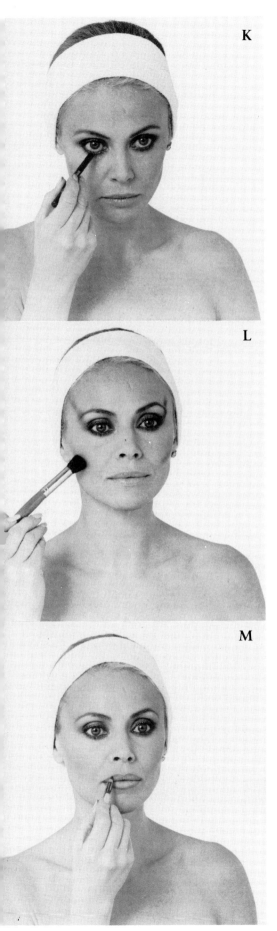

K

L

M

beginning of my make-up routine – which helps stop the colour bleeding – my technique is to outline with a medium-toned lip pencil (nothing too dark, I don't like that 'lipliner lady' look) (**M**), then to take a little Indian Earth and rub it over my lips. It's a good, gentle colour. Then I use gloss: either my good old Eight Hour Cream again or a Max Factor gloss in a pot or a Lancôme gloss in a stick. Either way, I choose the hardest consistency I can find. Roll-on glosses usually only last five minutes.

As alternatives to the Indian Earth I use something pale pink or perhaps an apricot shade. I also like a touch of Estée Lauder's gold lipstick which is like adding metallic glow. Unless you've got black hair – in which case you can go crazy with bright red Spanish dancer-type lips – I'd stick with light beige colours or colour glosses.

If you've got big lips like me, obviously you should never go outside the natural lipline or you will look like one big walking lip. Frankly, even if you have thin lips, I wouldn't recommend going outside the natural lipline. It just doesn't work. What happens is that you eat off the centre, leaving a false ring round the edge of your mouth.

---

* Contrary to popular belief, it's OK to use a borrowed comb or brush – few adults have head lice these days – but never lend or borrow your eye make-up implements, brushes, sponges, lipsticks or blushers. If someone asks you in the Ladies room, the answer should always be a firm, if rude, no.
* Clean make-up brushes weekly in mild soap and water. Dry naturally, handle down in a glass. You can disinfect them by dipping the bristles only into alcohol. Shake well after.
* Sharpen pencils weekly whether they need it or not. It keeps the tips clean and free of bacteria.

I've been a brunette and a redhead, but this make-up still works well with any colouring. I wore a brunette wig in the TV movie *Valley of the Dolls* – actually it was Jackie Bisset's wig from *Rich and Famous* – they were economizing! I went red for *The Night They Raided Minsky's* – not blazing, flaming red, more of a strawberry-ish colour. The make-up stays the same but if you're a brunette you might add slightly stronger eyebrows, a little stronger blush. During the summer or when you have a tan, go easy on the powders and favour the shiny look which enhances it.

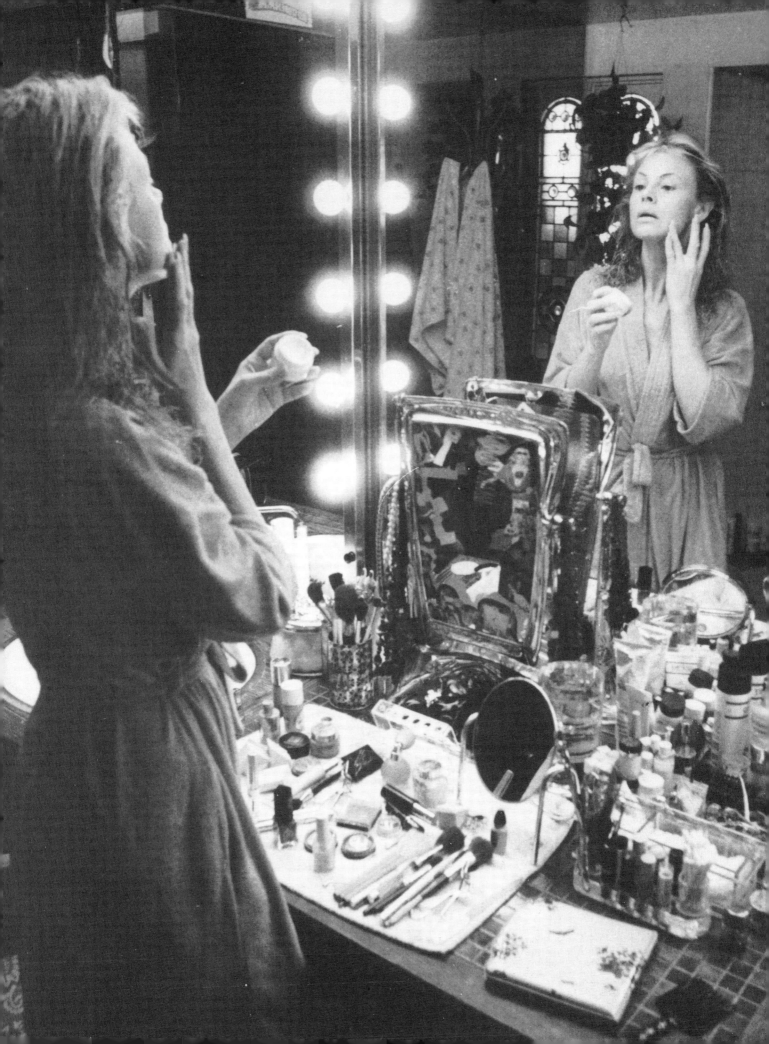

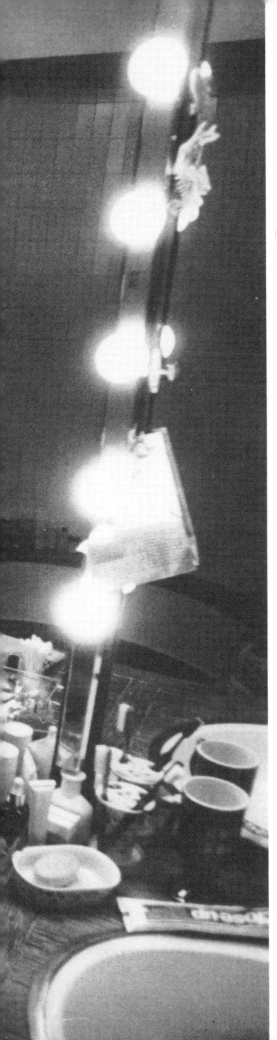

Seeing Yourself in the Right Light

Stand as far away from your make-up mirror as your eyesight will allow. That is how most people are going to see you and that is the view you are interested in. Obviously you can't put on mascara from ten miles away, but other than that there's no need to press your nose against the mirror.

Make up in the right light. If you make up in a brightly lit bathroom and then go out into daylight, you might get quite a different picture of yourself if you checked your make-up again in a mirror outdoors. That's how women end up with horrific blobs of rouge or foundation stripes at the jawline. Ideally you should make up in the exact light you expect to be in: daylight for daytime, and artificial light for evenings.

Useful Tips

If Your Eyes are Smallish or Close Together. . .
Concentrate your eye make-up on the outer half of your eye only. It visually sets your eyes wider apart. Avoid ringing them with a dark pencil or kohl, which will only make them look beadier than ever.

If My Make-up Has to Last the Whole Day. . .
I 'fix' it with Evian spray. Before the mascara and lipstick go on, I hold the atomizer far away from my face and squirt a very light mist over my whole face. Keep it very light, needless to say, otherwise your make-up will run. If necessary I gently pat it dry with a tissue – never rub – but if you spray lightly it should dry naturally within a few seconds.

The Indian Earth Trick
When you are tanned, Indian Earth is a great face shaper to make your face look smaller. You can draw it round the edges of your face like a mask – across the top of your forehead under your fringe, if you have one, down the cheekbones, around the jawbone. Blend well, of course.

Make-up Sense
Amidst the confusion of products seducing you from the make-up counters, you won't waste your money if you stick to powders in all your buys. They stay put longer and look softer, smoother and much more professional. You can touch up forever with powders.

Ready to Go
I keep my make-up laid out on a towel or cover a table with Kleenex or kitchen roll. I use it to dab off excess powder from my brushes and change it as soon as it looks grimy.

Cold Comfort

Red noses glow in the dark from a great distance and look highly unattractive. The best possible camouflage for a cold, red Rudolph nose is of course a permanent suntan.

But realistically speaking, if you live in a cold climate and constantly have to cope with a miserable, blue look, start with lots and lots of moisturizer. I would opt for a heavier one than usual, that is less likely to sink straight in without trace. The idea is to leave some kind of moist barrier on your skin.

Foundation is an absolute must – keep it handy in your make-up bag and remember to touch up when you've blown your nose. It's the only way to conceal that glowing red hooter. Don't use a camouflage stick because they are too drying and you will end up with a flaky-looking skin.

Choose a foundation shade a touch darker than usual. A tan shade works better than a pale, whitish one since it helps kill the blue tones in your skin.

Avoid powder at all costs. It will return your skin to its dry state in a flash. On the ski slopes is the one time I favour cream blush which stays put better and makes my skin look less dry.

Spot Check

I'm very lucky, touch wood, and not the pimply type, but once in a while when I have my period I'll get one. My daughter used to have problems with her skin but they've disappeared since she gave up junk foods. Chapter 3 tells you how to get rid of spots, but first you'll need to cover the little beasts with a concealer stick or pencil. It's more hygienic to dab it on to your finger and then pat it on to your pimple. Use a clean finger every time and wash your hands well afterwards. That way you minimize the chance of infecting the skin around it.

Powder over, using a cotton wool ball which you throw out immediately. Next dab on a touch of make-up base and re-powder.

Keep the cover-stick handy so you can touch up during the day when it rears its ugly little head again, as it will undoubtedly do. Do not despair. It's unlikely to last more than a couple of days.

If you're going to wear a bare, strappy dress, check that you haven't got a big unsightly blemish on your shoulders. If you have, cover it up with concealer stick using the same method. You wouldn't ignore it if it was on your face.

In the Mood to Sparkle?

I love the excitement of getting ready for a party – to me it's half the fun deciding what to wear, trying on different dresses and showing them to the kids, swapping ideas with girlfriends or, if I am going with a man, perhaps deciding we will both go wearing black, for instance. It's fun, too, to spend the afternoon relaxing in the hairdressers and maybe getting them to try something a little unusual or to put a decoration in my hair. To my mind, if your hosts are going to the trouble of throwing a great party, the least you can do is go to the same amount of trouble to look terrific and get in the right mood.

Allow plenty of time to get ready. There's no point in flinging yourself in the shower and rushing out of the house with damp hair, or going to your drawer only to find the only black tights you possess are sporting a great big ladder.

On the other hand, you don't want to be ready two hours ahead of time because you'll find yourself fidgeting and fiddling, putting on more make-up and wishing you hadn't and playing around with your hair until it looks greasy.

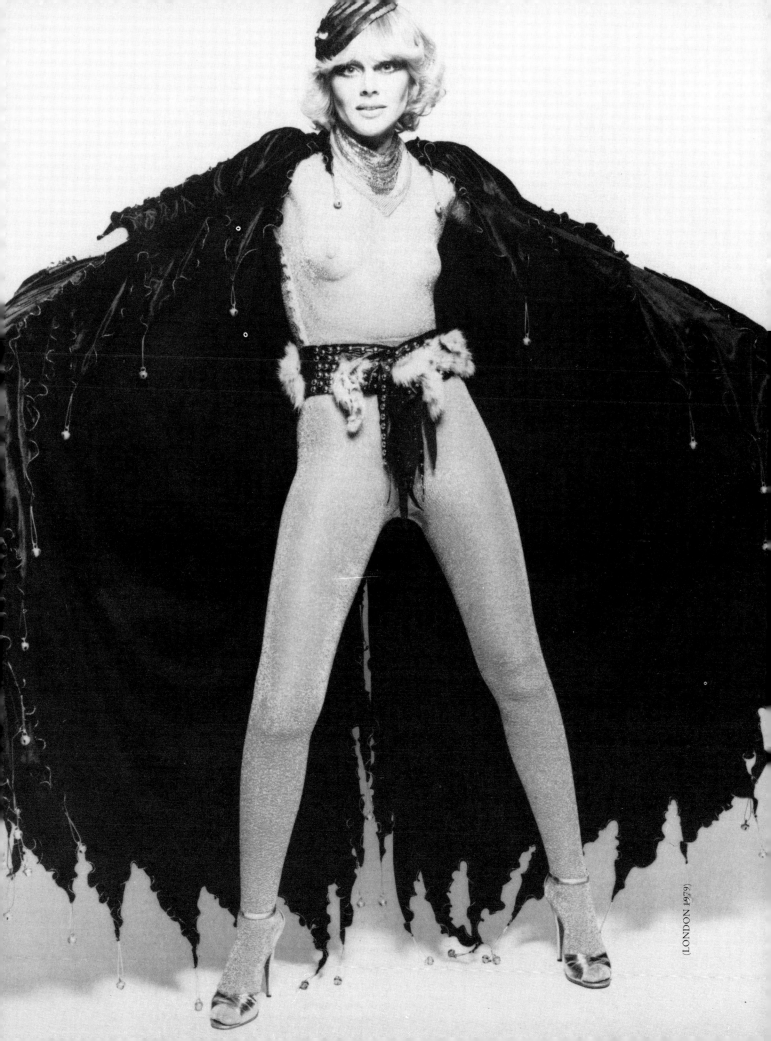

(LONDON 1979)

Try to time it right, particularly if you need to wind down from the day. Lay all your alternative outfits out on the bed, along with shoes and tights to match.

I give myself a face mask to get in the mood, and maybe use a collagen ampoule. If you can find it, try a little Marylin Miglin Pheromone body lotion, it's fabulously scented and shimmering. If not, look for something with the same effect. Glittery body powders aren't such a clever idea since they come off on everything you wear and the glitter powder is almost impossible to get rid of.

Sparkly eye shadows – powder or gel – are another story, though, since you use so little of them and they're great fun to experiment with for evenings. Shimmery whites and golds look very glamorous if you just dust them over your browbone. Try a touch in the centre of your upper eyelid just above the lashes – that looks pretty too.

Taking It Off

I'm proud to say that I can still count the nights when I've collapsed into bed wearing my make-up. Unless I can't walk, I take it off.

Cleansers are the perfect example of a situation where I opt for a basic product rather than a famous name with fancy packaging. What is the point of paying the earth for something that's on and off your skin in two minutes and only lasts for a couple of weeks? Thank goodness cleansers have improved from the days of thick, gooey cold cream which took forever to wipe off. Today the rule is the lighter the better. And preferably non-perfumed.

The same goes for eye make-up remover. For years I couldn't read in bed because my eyes were all glued up with gook. You're looking for something not too greasy, and Estée Lauder make one that doesn't put me out of action.

If you use waterproof mascara, it's hell to get off and you're better off using mineral oil, baby oil or almond oil on a wet cotton wool pad. I only wear waterproof mascara if I want to look good in the pool or at the beach, or if I'm planning to go to bed with it on or have a tearful scene to do in a film. It does seem to turn your lashes into sharp spikes and somehow I can't believe that's good for them.

Mascara that can be removed with water is bound to be more gentle. You don't need to, but I still prefer to use a proper eye make-up remover on a cotton wool pad. I just rub gently with circular movements. I know we are told not to touch the delicate eye area, but how else can you get mascara off? You don't have to do your eyes like you do your kitchen floor, but you do have to rub.

Once my eyes are clean I put facial cleanser into the palm of my hand and massage it all over my face and neck. I wipe it off with a tissue. If you're stuck, you can always manage with oil instead – baby oil, coconut oil, almond oil or mineral oil work well.

My skin is basically normal so I don't need a strong skin toner and choose a non-alcohol type because it is less drying. If you've got an oily skin you'll fare better with a cleansing milk followed by an alcohol astringent.

Next I use Estée Lauder's Night Repair followed with a night-time moisturizer and rich eye cream and anti-wrinkle cream (see Chapter 3).

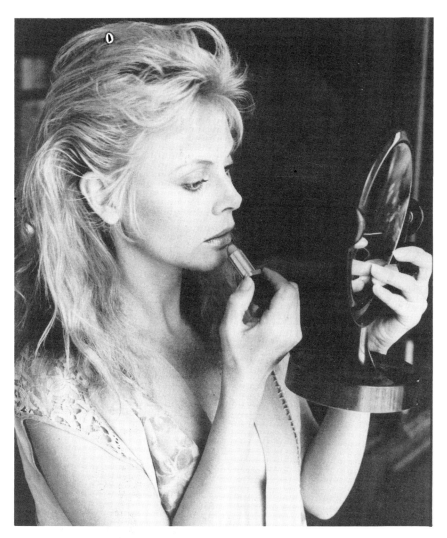

Make-up to go to Bed In

If you want to look your most sensual in the bedroom, the right make-up will certainly help. Hypo-allergenic make-up, like Max Factor's Swedish Formula or Clinique, is best for bedtime. Don't use dollops of foundation, just a light covering to conceal blemishes and even out the skin tone.

Choose a lighter colour than your usual daytime shade. You can even go a shade lighter than your skin colour if you wish because the dim bedroom lighting automatically makes your skin look darker, and the paler your skin the more your eyes will be enhanced, which is the object of the exercise.

For the same reason, mascara is more important than anything else. The waterproof kind is virtually sleep-proof and if a little does come off on your pillow, it's a small price to pay. Maybelline and Max Factor waterproof mascaras are good.

Use a little eye shadow all over your top lids. Ash brown looks the most natural and suits everybody, but you can use a slate grey if you prefer. I wouldn't bother with anything else. If all goes according to plan your cheeks will be naturally rouged up anyway! Powder is the main give-away clue that you are wearing make-up, so why use it?

Nothing is more sensual than the bedroom-eyed look, though, so put on the brown eye shadow and practise in front of the bathroom mirror.

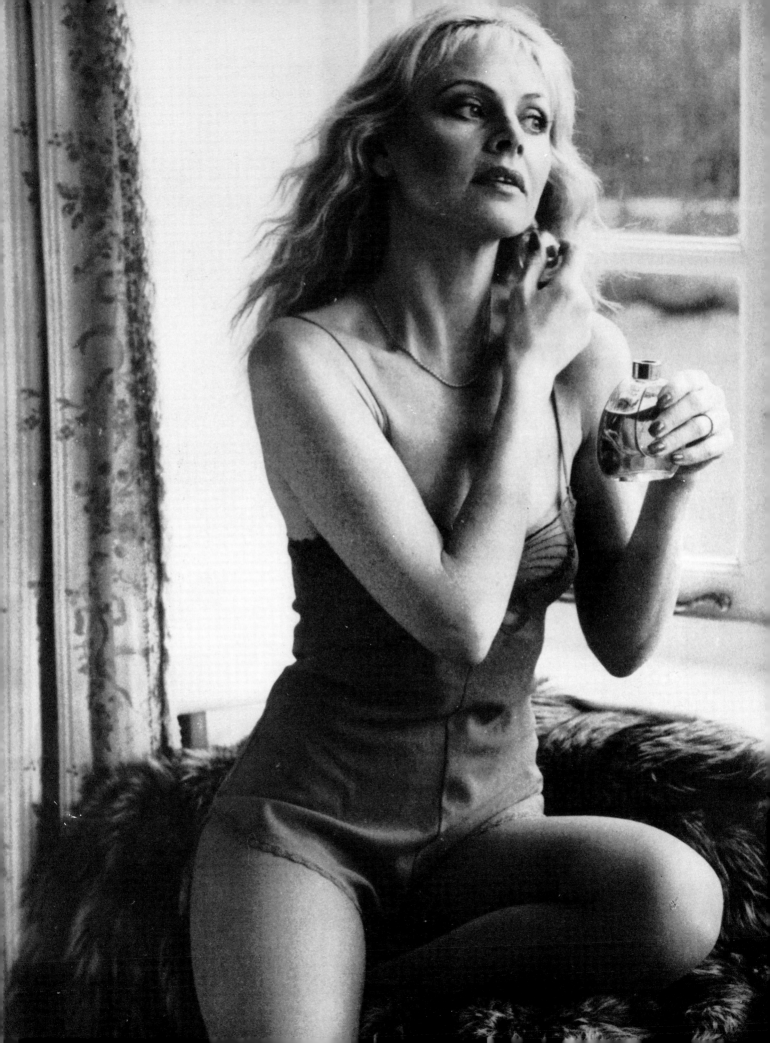

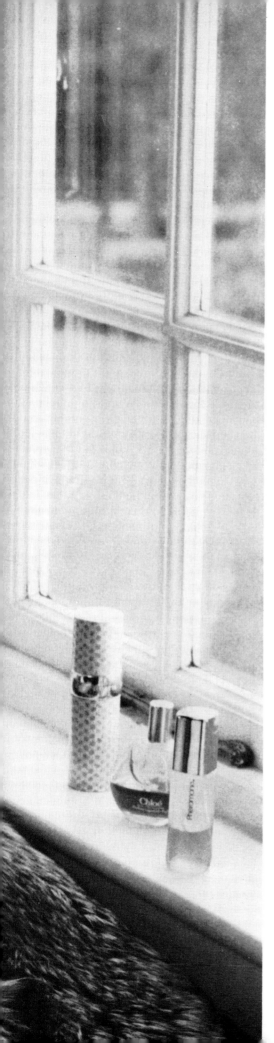

9/THE MYSTIQUE OF SCENT

Smell is an incredibly powerful sensual signal. We all have our own personal odour – and I'm not talking about stale sweat, or even fresh sweat for that matter – but the subtle, natural scents that draw a man to a woman and a woman to a man. Even scientists still can't fathom quite how it works, so what hope do we have? But what we do know is that smell is one of our most vital senses.

Animal experiments seem to have proved that our romantic instincts ebb and flow with the presence of smell. Apparently our brain's message systems can break down and analyse and respond to every individual scent. This can happen on two levels simultaneously, so if you get that little 'ping' in your head that says you fancy a man, the attraction can actually be in response to his natural body scent on one level *and* the aftershave he is wearing on another.

For me it is hard to beat the smell of clean, fresh skin, but nevertheless I love perfume. So do men. One man I knew always lavished me with gifts of Patou's Joy, which I hated, but I didn't have the heart to tell him. Sometimes you have to make concessions to keep a man happy, so I just wore it when we went out together. Men do seem to love Joy, but I suspect they like it not so much for the scent as for its aura of glamour – after all, it is the world's most expensive, exclusive perfume.

I find most men like light, refreshing perfumes and so do I. I would never buy cheap perfume, not through any kind of snobbery but because expensive perfumes contain natural floral oils and the real thing is distinctly more alluring than the synthetic substitutes which get used in the cheap brands. Joy, for instance, contains a rare Bulgarian rose and jasmine which is specially picked by hand in the early hours of the morning. Small wonder it's expensive.

Perfumes can be made with as few as six ingredients or as many as fifty or sixty, so you can see where the price variations come in. One of the most expensive components is the fixative, which is why pricier perfumes do tend to linger longer.

There's More to Buying than Meets the Nose

What smells like a million dollars on you might smell like cabbage on me. Perfume is so personal that I'd never try to recommend individual fragrances. You can talk about 'grassy top notes' and 'floral tones' until you are blue in the face, but there is no real way to convey a fragrance in words and there is absolutely no substitute for testing it yourself and working by trial and error until you find one you really love.

When buying perfume you have to remember that you are dealing with a complicated fusion of skin and bottled fragrance. The pH factor of your skin – which indicates how acid or alkaline it is – affects what happens to a scent on your skin. So does what you eat, apparently. And if you are a vegetarian, scientists say that you could unconsciously reject anything with an animal ingredient.

Of course we always talk about 'perfume', but the concentrated perfume isn't automatically the best choice over and above cologne or eau de toilette. For a start there's the price; secondly, your own sense of smell doesn't always correspond with other people's, so rather than assault them with half a bottle of perfume it is often better to play safe with a light spritz of cologne or eau de toilette. No one will find that offensive.

I like atomizers for precisely that reason. I don't use the purse-size ones, which don't last five minutes. If you want to carry fragrance with you, fill up those little trial-size bottles and keep the atomizer at home.

Never buy a perfume from a quick first impression. Always give it a good ten minutes to warm up on the inside of your wrist before you make a judgement. When you first put it on you get a whiff of what is known in the trade as the 'top notes'. These are often not the most attractive, tending to be sharper, and they are also the first to disappear. The real body of the perfume lingers, and you should base your decision on that.

To make the most of your perfume, apart from dabbing it behind your ears in the traditional fashion, try putting it on all the places where you naturally sweat. You know what happens to your body when you exercise – sweat trickles between your breasts, inside your arms, down your back, and in the creases between your legs. Those are the body's natural hot spots that will make the fragrance waft up.

---

* Never use so-called 'feminine hygiene' sprays and never use perfume on your private parts, only ever in the creases of flesh at the tops of your thighs.

It's fun to have a whole host of perfumes, but since they linger in your clothes – unless you wash them after each wearing – it doesn't make great sense to chop and change and end up with an awful pong.

I like my clothes to be totally individual and different from everyone else's, but with perfume all that matters is that I like it. Frankly it doesn't bother me if five hundred people are wearing the same one. Guerlain's Shalimar is my special favourite, but I also love Yves St Laurent's Opium and the classic Bal à Versailles – three scents which, if they should linger in my wardrobe, blend without clashing.

It's important to give your perfume a chance to do its job properly. Don't overload yourself with competitive scents from, say, deodorant, talc, soap, and hairspray. Deodorant and hairspray tend to have very strong whiffs and the concoction of odours from that little lot could be enough to send any man rushing for fresh air!

I make a point of buying everything unperfumed except for perfume. What you can also do, of course, is have everything to match. I love getting a gift of my perfume in soap or shampoo, and when Christmas or my birthday come around I drop big hints to my kids since those are things I rarely buy for myself.

To be told that your body smells terrific is one of the highest compliments you can be paid.

Now a couple of practical tips with sensuality in mind.

A Breath Of Fresh Air

Whatever I wear, I hang it outside for at least twenty-four hours for a good airing before I put it back in my wardrobe. I'm lucky because I've got a covered balcony in Los Angeles and a garden in London. If you haven't got an outside spot, hang clothes in your bathroom and turn the shower on for a little bit of steam. Give them a good shake and leave them hanging for a couple of hours before you put them away.

I don't have a saintly attitude about smoking – I smoked myself from the time I was fifteen until I was twenty-eight – but I can't stand the smell of stale cigarette smoke in clothes. Victoria has stopped smoking now, but when she was puffing away I thought I was going to die every time I opened her wardrobe. When she stopped I hung everything outside for a whole week.

I don't mind people smoking in my home because I don't think you can allow yourself the luxury of telling other people what to do – but you can ban smoking in the bedroom, that seems fair.

In Praise Of Pot Pourri

I put big bowls of it in my wardrobes and shoe cupboards, even the cupboard that I keep my handbags in. I don't put it in with my undies though, somehow I think the smell is too strong for one's knickers! Besides, that part of the body is super-sensitive anyway and as long as everything is clean, I just don't think they need pot-pourriing!

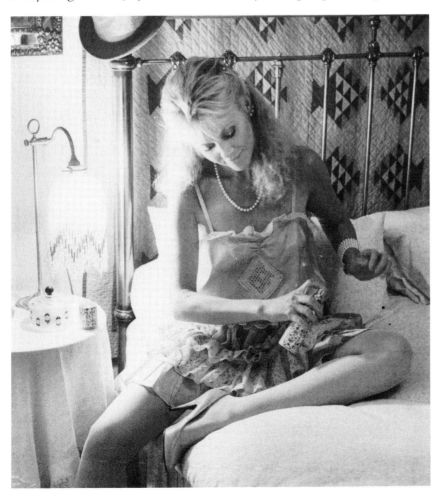

10 / EATING FOR A SENSUAL LIFE

I rarely need to see a doctor. I firmly believe that if you eat well and take good care of your body, you will stay healthy. The bonus is that you will also keep your weight down and that is vital to feeling sensual.

Like many people I was brought up by a caring mother who fed me good-quality food but left me a legacy of misconceptions that took years to break down – false notions like 'Your body needs three meals a day' and 'Sweeties are a reward for being a good girl.' I know that I can quite easily live on two small meals a day. You should consult your doctor before you drastically change your diet, but three meals a day are, I think, unnecessary. Far from falling apart, my body looks better than ever.

You can choose to be fat or slim, agile or stiff, taut or flabby. Make no mistake about it, your body's fate lies in your own hands. I'm not a paragon of virtue, doling out rules and regulations, and I've committed various major sins against my own body. I'm not saying 'Don't eat in French restaurants', 'Don't eat fatty foods', and 'Don't drink'. I am all for the 'eat, drink and be merry' philosophy but everything carries a price tag and you can't continually abuse yourself without doing some repair work. If I abuse my car the clutch will wear out. If I don't get it serviced it will break down. Why should my body be any different?

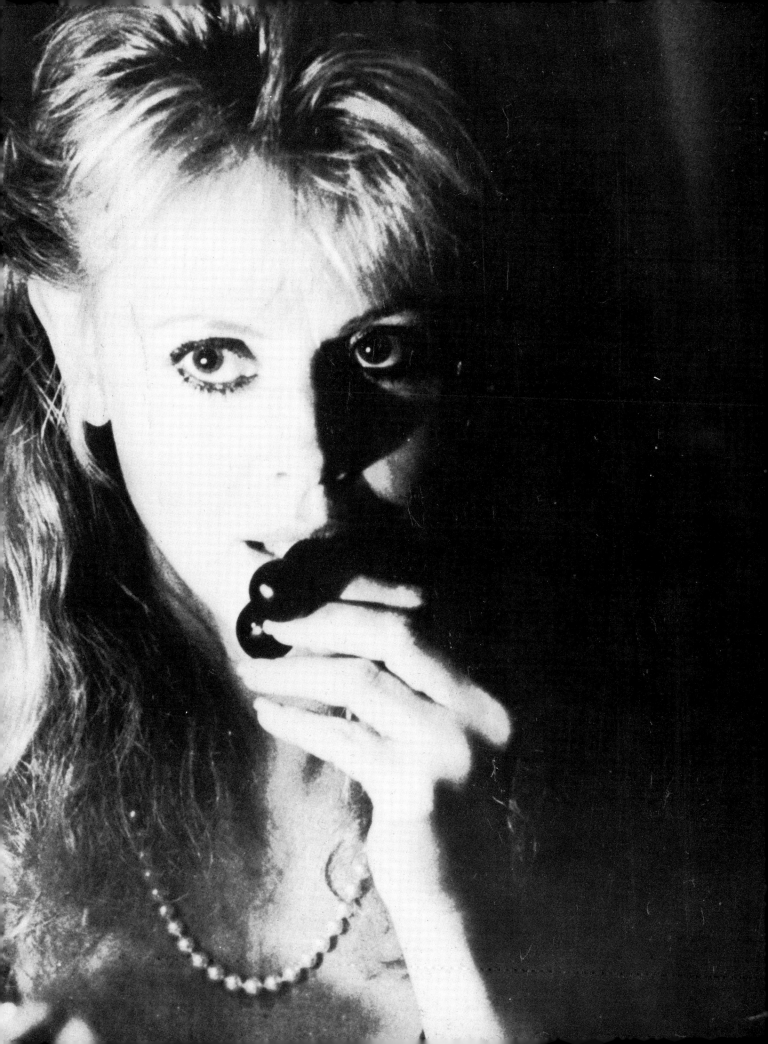

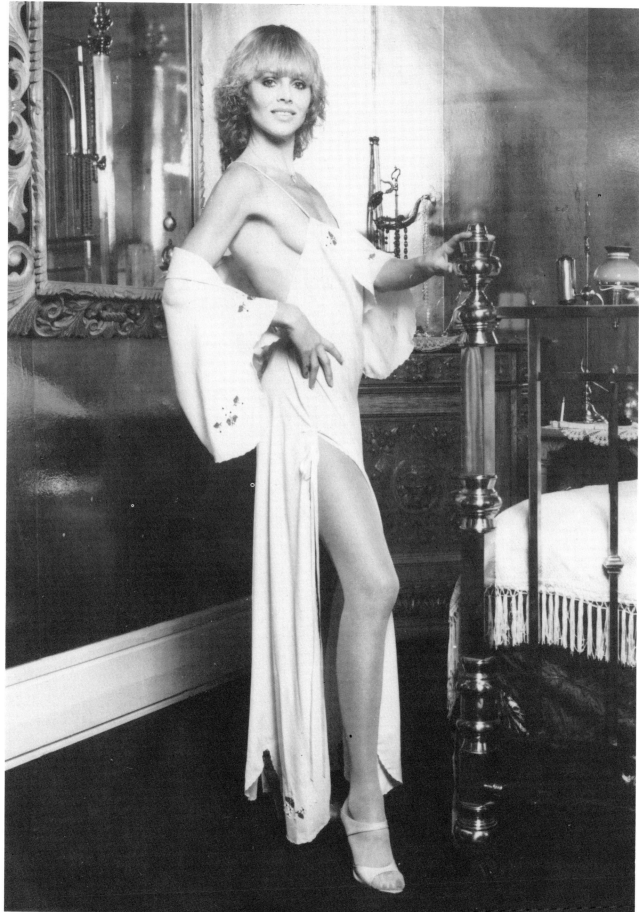

(LONDON 1978)

There are hundreds of books on the subject of diet and health that you can read to get a better understanding of your body – I'm concerned here only with the sensual aspects of eating.

Food itself, after all, can be very sensual – big, plump, black grapes with no pips; firm, furry kiwi fruits reminiscent of a certain piece of male anatomy, yet green and succulent inside. Strawberries and raspberries are sensual because they feel as though they are dissolving in your mouth. Apples are not sensual, despite Eve. Nor are any foods you have to chomp on. Chomping and crunching aren't sensual . . . sucking is.

Over-indulgence isn't sensual. Nor is bingeing. A light meal that tantalizes your tastebuds yet doesn't entirely satisfy your appetite – now that *is* sensual. It's also conducive to lovemaking.

If you've stuffed yourself full of pasta, your mind is more likely to be filled with thoughts of indigestion tablets than erotic fantasies. If you've washed the pasta down with a bottle of heavy wine you're probably counting the minutes until you can collapse into bed, to sleep but not to have sex. There's nothing sensual about a heavy tum nor the rolls of flesh that result from it.

What you eat can and does have a fairly immediate effect on your mood and how you feel about yourself. A long, lingering meal can be very sensual. I'd favour light white wine or champagne in preference to red which makes your mouth feel and taste stale. Take the dessert into the bedroom and finish it off after lovemaking for a double sensual treat.

Assess Yourself

Strip off in front of a mirror and ask yourself if what you see is a pretty sight. Unless you're a ballet dancer or a gymnast, ninety-eight times out of a hundred it is not. If you want to lose weight and have a slim, beautiful body, corny as it may sound, start with your mind.

Ultimately all diets work. What fails is people's ability to stick to them and that's why attitude is so important. There may be times when you just can't seem to lose weight, no matter what you do, but it's probably because you are not committed enough. Losing weight starts in your head, nowhere else. The evidence that you need to lose weight may be on your bum and thighs but the actual desire and decision lies in your head. Keep repeating to yourself; 'I do want to be thin', 'I do want to lose weight', 'I do want to look great in a bikini.'

When your body has picked up all these signals and you are truly ready, the next step is obvious: **EAT LESS!** Initially you are bound to feel deprived. It's like being used to a lot of sex. If suddenly it's not there, you want it and you think about it all the time. But, except for nymphomaniacs, the less you have the less you want. It's the same with food. The less food you put into your body, the less food your body is going to crave.

I believe goals are vital. I wanted to be thin for my fortieth birthday. I also wanted to be rich and I would have liked to have been married and to have had another child. I didn't achieve all of those things. But I was thin, so one out of four isn't bad.

Food Confessions

I wasn't born with a bottomless pit of willpower. On a naughty night I've been known to tuck away chicken and green beans – a nice low calorie meal – and to follow it up by a cheese sandwich, an apple and a Mars bar! Still not satisfied, I've filled up with cheesecake or something chocolatey or custard-filled, with a couple of dozen licorice twists to finish off. . . .

When I was pregnant with Victoria, things got worse. No one said, 'Don't eat for two, it doesn't work that way.' I was married and living in the country, with only the local tuck shop for amusement. Those little country houses are all very well, with their antiques and log fires, but what the hell do you do all day? I ate. Boredom makes you hungry and, thanks to the tuck shop's bottomless pit of Mars bars and my other eating indulgences, I put on 42 lb. It was gross – I met the sides of the bathtub. Victoria was tiny, weighing 5 lb 10 oz when she was born, so I can't blame her.

I'd also stopped smoking, and I had a doting husband in Sellers who was nineteen years my senior and really didn't care how large I was as long as I was young and had long, blonde hair.

I think I had heartburn every hour of the day. My last supper before I gave birth gives you a clue to my eating patterns. It was an enormous Chinese meal guzzled down in our suite at the Dorchester in London.

Overeating is depressing, not just psychologically but physically. Some foods are more depressing than others. Foods high in carbohydrates, for instance, tend to lie heavily in your stomach and if you feel like a blob the chances are you will look like one too. You will project a 'blobbie' attitude and that's not sensual.

Sugar is particularly dangerous. Like all 'empty' carbohydrates it gives you a shot of false energy, a high. Not only does the high disappear with a crash, but the thought of the damage you've done to your weight is also depressing. Worse still, sugar unfortunately stimulates the desire for more sugar, which is why I won't keep sweets in the house, nor biscuits or cake. If you have a taste, you want more.

Today I rarely order a dessert, even in a very good restaurant. I don't need it and I liken it to opening a door. Once you open the door you let all the little devils in so it's better not to open it. Be satisfied with a good dinner and turn down the free after-dinner mint. Think of yourself as an alcoholic or a junkie and give your particular weakness a wide berth.

If you want to indulge occasionally, I recommend hiding a few of the finest chocolates in your deep freeze – that way you can't bite into them immediately but have to defrost first. If you are determined to 'sin', then at least it will be for something fabulous.

Mind you, I don't believe in guilt. If you are going to pig out – and there are days when we all fall from the straight and narrow – then do it, enjoy it and get back on the track tomorrow. Once you have made your decision, feeling guilty is futile.

For years I've followed a healthy eating pattern, understood it and found it quite easy – boring, but relatively easy. But days still dawn when my whole new attitude disappears down the drain and I undo all my good work for something as silly as chocolate-covered peanuts. It's never worth it, but that doesn't stop me.

I have given up meat, cigarettes, coffee, and all alcohol except for the odd beer. They didn't leave my life with a cry and a whimper – it was more like a bang. I'm an impulsive person, it's all or nothing. One morning I woke up and said, 'I'm never going to smoke again.' Something just snapped. There's nothing sensual about puffing on a cigarette and there's certainly nothing sensual about tobacco breath. I gave up meat the same way. Meat made me feel sluggish and red meat tends to be fatty and high in calories, so I believe it was a healthy decision.

Coffee was a tough one. There's nothing in the world to me like Swedish coffee and I was the ultimate coffee lover. Yet one day in April 1982 I said 'That's it', and I haven't tasted it since.

I know coffee has been accused of contributing to hypertensive heart disease, not to mention the possible link between coffee and cancer of the bladder and the lower urinary tract, but I don't think that was what did it. Coffee is an artificial stimulant: it makes me red in the face and nervous, and I just made an out-of-the-blue overnight decision that I didn't need it any more.

Alcohol was a different story. My British driving licence was revoked because I was stopped by the police and found to have too much alcohol in my bloodstream. I wasn't drunk. In fact I had so little over the legal limit that when my mechanic picked up my car to store it for the year he laughed out loud. Nevertheless it was too much and they took my licence. The emotional shock of being put in a paddy wagon, placed in a solitary little room and questioned like a criminal was just too much for me. I think the shock and horror of that night stopped me drinking and since 10 June 1982 nothing but beer has passed my lips.

It was a very traumatic time. I didn't stop drinking to punish myself, I just stopped. That October my daughter Victoria threw a surprise birthday party for me and insisted that I greet my friends with Dom Pérignon. I took one mouthful and let it run back into the glass, it tasted so foul. I've been on a private aircraft since then where they were serving nothing but Kristal Brut. I've been at dinner parties where pink Taittinger was flowing like milk from a mother's breast, but I just don't have the taste for it any more and I'm glad. Pink skin and bloodshot eyes are hardly sensual and they are definite by-products of drinking alcohol. So are dry, black-tinged lips and sour breath, not to mention the facial bloat.

Baby sweets, licorice and real kiddie foods are my downfall. And although I know for a fact I will never drink wine or champagne again, I can't truthfully say that I will never eat another sweet. My mind hasn't made that decision yet.

I have a rule about salt and sugar. I never mix them. They don't agree, which is why the day after you eat them you may resemble a balloon about to burst and your eyes are probably puffy.

As an actress I long ago vowed never to eat Chinese food or any salty food, or drink wine or eat cake, the night before filming. I know I'm going to wake up bloated in my face and body and I also know it could take twenty-four hours to disappear.

Eat Chinese food by all means, but stick to beer or, better still, mineral water. No sweet soda obviously, and I personally would never touch the diet stuff – you might as well buy a bottle of artificial colouring.

Salty foods like caviar are distinctly unsexy. They leave you dry-mouthed and thirsty, neither of which enhances the way you kiss.

Eating healthily will ensure you have the stamina for all those long nights of lovemaking. Stay away from crisps and dips, processed foods, tinned products, and fizzy drinks. Give sweets, cakes, bread, and biscuits a miss. Help yourself to light, fresh foods like fruit and vegetables.

Cut down on alcohol. Just remind yourself that it can destroy brain cells and stop your liver processing fat, and that just four drinks a day are enough to cause organ damage. At the very least it will dehydrate you, dry out your skin, and keep you tossing and turning at night. Doesn't sound very sexy, does it? If you must have the odd glass of wine, dilute it with soda.

I happen not to believe in cellulite. But I do know that women are prone to ugly, dimpled fat in their nether regions and there is nothing very sensual about it. I believe in treating dairy foods with caution. Milk, butter, cheese, cottage cheese, and yogurt are mucus-forming and should only be eaten in strict moderation. Has it ever come to your attention that there is a striking resemblance between cottage cheese and that wobbly fat padding out your thighs?

Dr Bieler's Miracle Anti-bloat Broth

If I do ever find myself with that puffy bloat, I swear by Dr Bieler's broth – it's a combination of four vegetables that make the perfect mineral-potassium blend for your body. It's basically a liver and kidney cleanser and if you start on it at eight in the morning, I can almost guarantee you will look pretty good by eight that night. And your skin will look wonderful.

To make the broth chop up some zucchini (courgettes), green beans, celery, and parsley into four equal-sized piles. Start cooking the harder vegetables first in a pint of water, so give the celery and green beans a five-minute lead, then add the rest and simmer the whole lot for twenty minutes. Let the broth cool a bit, then whoosh it up in your blender. It might look rather disgusting but in my opinion it's delicious. Store it in the fridge. It's best to eat the broth plain, but if you feel so inclined you can add a herb of your choice. I'm very partial to dill, but tarragon, rosemary, and oregano are good. No salt and pepper.

This is the routine I follow for one, two or three days, depending upon how strong my willpower is. If your eating habits include munching luncheon meat sandwiches, hot dogs and sugar pops, this is going to come as a shock to you!

Start the day with just plain water or herb tea. Mint tea is best if you're totally unused to herb teas, since it's a familiar taste. No sugar or sweetener in the tea.

Then have a good bowlful of Bieler broth, hot or cold, whichever you prefer. You can eat as much of the broth as you like throughout the day, and drink as much herb tea as you want, plus a minimum of eight glasses of water. That's it for the day.

Ideally, keep it up for three days. It's difficult, but the benefits are so immediate and gratifying and you will feel so beautifully slim that you won't dream of putting anything junky into your system again.

I usually manage two days, but even one day is worthwhile. The difference is, I find, incredible. In the days when I was still drinking wine and champagne I might start a movie on a Friday with a puffy face. Over the weekend I would take myself in hand and rush to the Bieler broth. By Monday morning no one could believe the difference in me.

Be Kind to Your Insides

There's nothing romantic about an attack of indigestion, or worse still, wind or an upset tummy. Unless you are that extraordinary metal-eating Frenchman whose digestive juices somehow manage to break down supermarket trolleys and bicycle handlebars, it pays to spare a thought for your poor digestive system.

I know we are brought up not to discuss such delicate matters, but just between the pages of this book let's try to face the fact that what goes up must come down, and what goes in must come out. A nut which you've chomped into four pieces will travel through your 30 feet

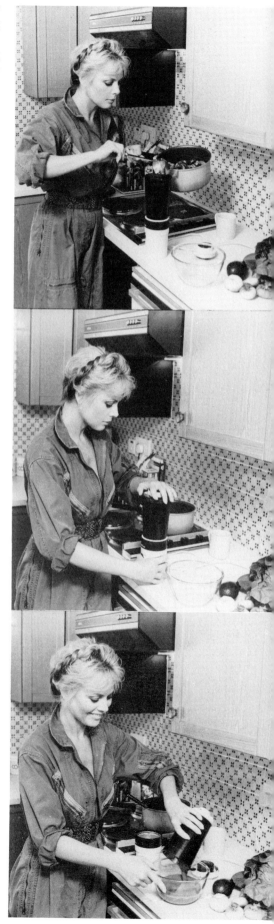

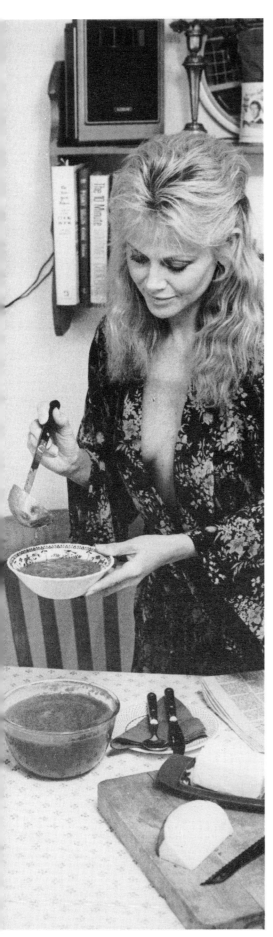

or so of digestive tract and upwards of fifteen hours later it will leave no doubt in the same four pieces, but minus the oils that your system has absorbed. Most of us just can't digest nuts.

There are definite repeat offenders – green and red peppers, onions, apple peel, tomato skin etc., but digestion is a personal matter and it's up to you to find your own list of no-nos.

I have trouble with salads in general, but particularly with that crunchy, watery lettuce that America produces, so I stick to the softer, leafy European kind. I know the crunchy stuff makes me suffer and I'm no fool. For no apparent reason I find I cannot eat green peppers, cooked or raw. To me they are indigestible and the same goes for broccoli, cauliflower, and huge amounts of garlic.

If you throw a goulash down your throat, it's nice to be able to anticipate the possible repercussions and make up your own mind if you want to suffer. Separate the ingredients in your mind. Decide what your particular body at your particular age can and can't digest.

Britt's Indigestion Cure (None of Us Is Perfect)
Empty out a headache or vitamin capsule and throw away the contents. Fill the capsule with powdered ginger from your kitchen shaker. Swallow it with a glass of cold water. Once it's down, drink a glass of warm water to help it dissolve fast. Give it a few minutes to travel through your miles of inner tubing, and nine times out of ten the indigestion will disappear.

Vitamin Cocktail

I swear that the vitamin and mineral supplements I take help give me boundless energy. While medical opinion varies on just what we should take and in what quantities, here is the daily dose that works for me.

I take at breakfast a fresh whole lemon squeezed into a 10oz glass of hot water; two big cups of tea with skim milk; a low-calorie yogurt; and a bowl of muesli or other cereal. Then I take my vitamin C: 5,000 or 6,000 mg daily if I'm in a cold climate, or 2,000 if I'm somewhere warm. I take the same amount later in the day to compensate for what whizzes through my system and out the other end! Vitamin C fights infection.

Some doctors will no doubt scream, but I take between 800 and 12,000 i.u. of vitamin E in dry form using the higher dosage when I have my period.

I take a very high-potency B complex pill (very important for hair, skin and eyes) and always check the labels before I buy to compare the mg content – some are better value than others. Invariably I buy a complex that has all the Bs combined with minerals but if not, I take those separately, buying high-potency, chelated minerals and doubling the suggested dose.

It can be dangerous to overdo vitamins A and D, but vitamin A is very good for your skin so I do take it daily. I take 25,000 i.u. and always take it in conjunction with vitamin E.

Wash vitamins down with plenty of water so they don't get stuck in the digestive tract and make you keep burping and honking. That's one advantage of fizzy vitamin C tablets (Redoxon), by the way – you dissolve them in water and drink them down.

A week before my period and during my period I take organic iron tablets as directed on the bottle, but I stop when my period is over.

Your body can only assimilate vitamins along with other foods and minerals, so always take them after a protein meal, preferably in the morning, but if your only main meal is late at night that's when you should take them.

Late-night Eating

Food is the fuel that drives your body through the day — why stoke the engines at night when you should be resting? What's more, late-night eating will make it tough for you to get a good night's sleep.

If you've eaten sweets or chocolate before going to bed you will have a particularly fitful time of it. It goes without saying that coffee has the same effect.

If you know you're going to be stuck with an unavoidably late dinner, have a big mug of low-calorie soup before you go out. It's a good idea to put something warm into your body like bouillon or consommé. I love the Japanese miso soup. It's a bit salty, but since I don't eat salt with anything else I live with that, and it's low in calories.

I learned the soup trick from years of late night premieres, but do it any time you suspect you'll be faced with endless cocktails and speeches before the food arrives.

When the food does appear, assuming it's the usual set menu, I always eat half-portions. I pick around anything I know my body can't digest easily. I don't care if my neighbours look at me in horror and nor should you.

If you do anticipate a fidgety night, try taking between six and ten calcium tablets with a glass of milk or a cup of camomile tea. That usually does the trick for me.

Take a Deep Breath

Ask yourself if you are guilty of exhaling fumes over those poor unfortunates around you? It goes without saying that you should avoid close encounters with garlic, onions, leeks, curries, or anything highly spiced if you are planning to snuggle up to someone. Red wine, cheeses, and even sweets are also culprits. Stick to nice, bland food, even if it is ever so tempting to chomp into that pickled onion. If I'm filming a love scene I always brush my teeth for good measure.

You should be particularly careful when you are dieting. When you are cleansing your body all the bad stuff comes out of you and you will probably notice that your tongue gets a coating on it. Some women have that problem when they have their period, but of course that's a very temporary state of affairs.

Unless you are urgently in need of a trip to the dentist and your mouth is one great, gaping cavity, breath troubles usually stem from tummy trouble like constipation or indigestion, or imperfectly cleaned teeth (see Chapter 6).

I do have friends who suffer from bad breath, and I must admit that for all my honesty I do find it hard to say anything. But if you live with someone, hopefully you'll come to the point where you'll feel free to talk openly if your breath is a little 'off colour'; but with a good diet and a clean mouth your breath should be naturally fresh.

I know it sounds horrid, but chewing on a sprig of parsley is a real cure-all. Or try one of those breath freshener sprays like Binaca — it's not as if you use them by the gallon, so just this once we can afford to overlook their sugar content. Let's face it, you have to love someone an awful lot to approach Dracula breath.

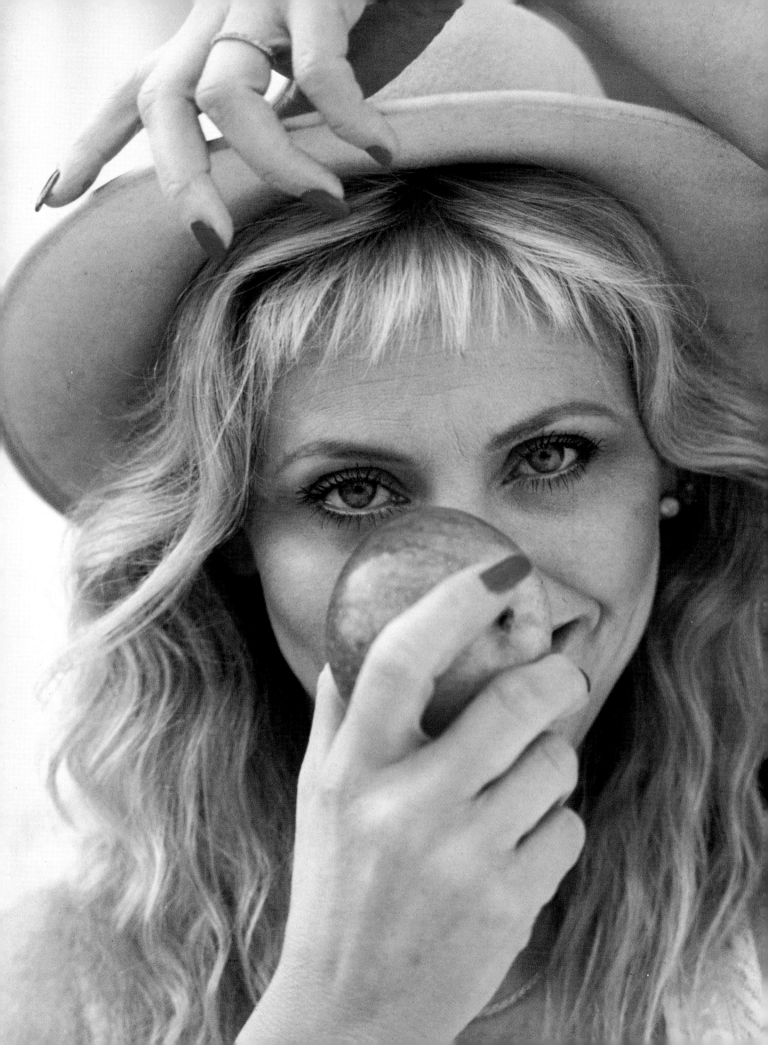

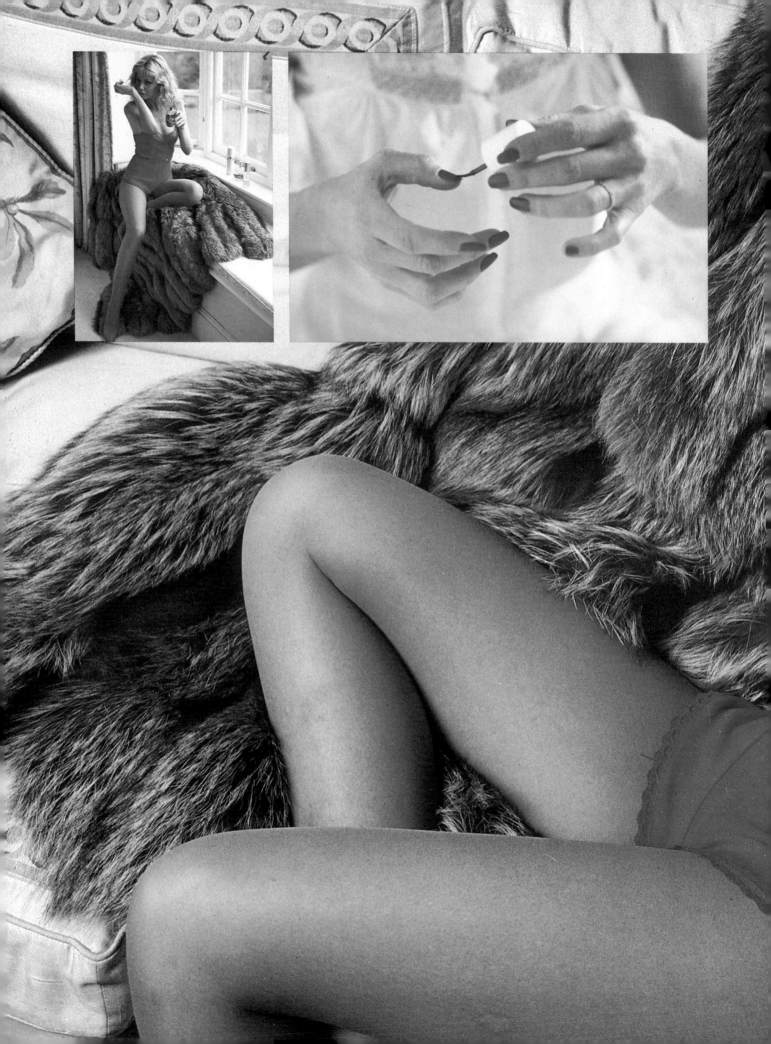

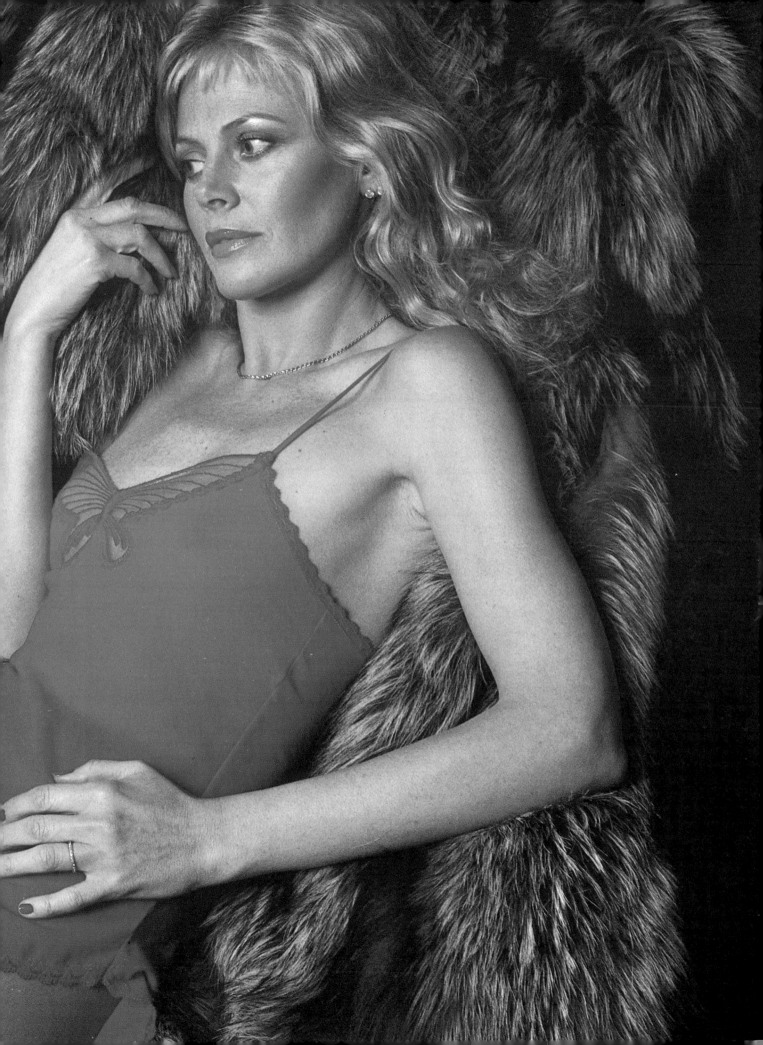

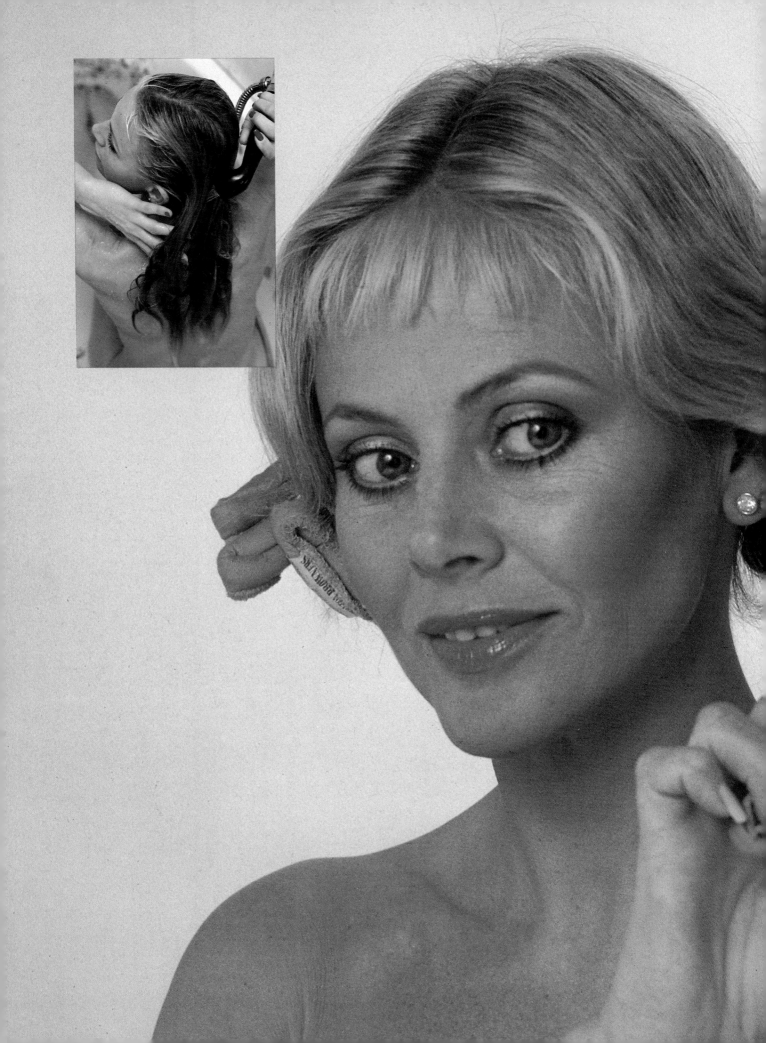

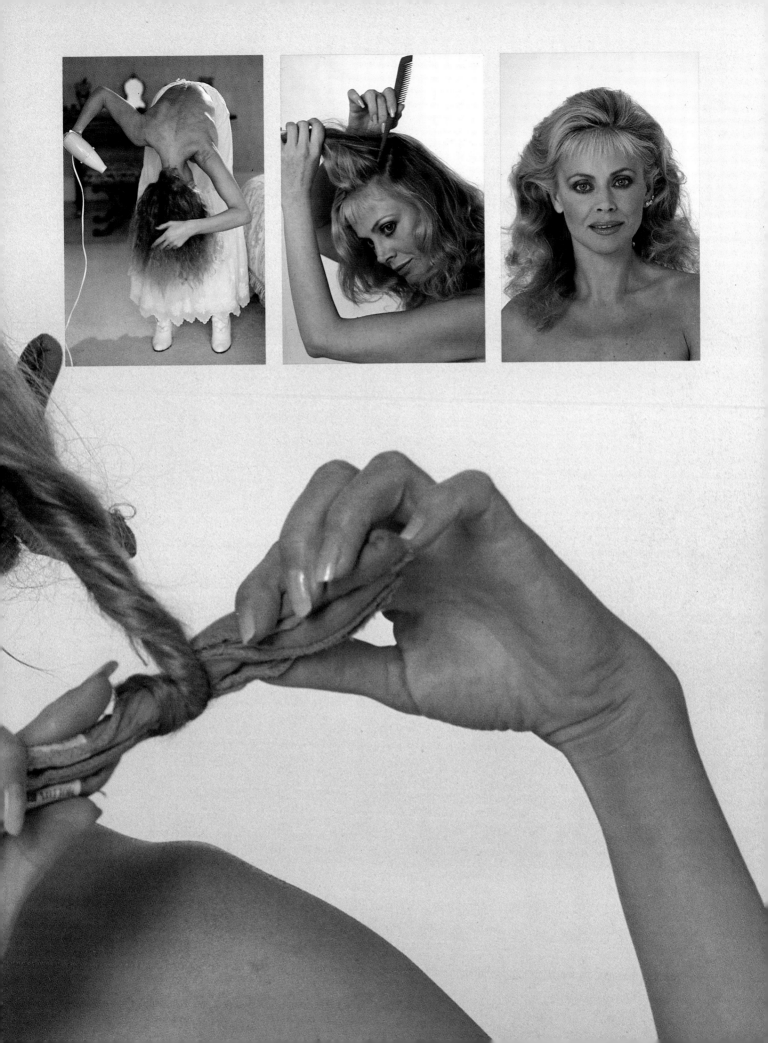

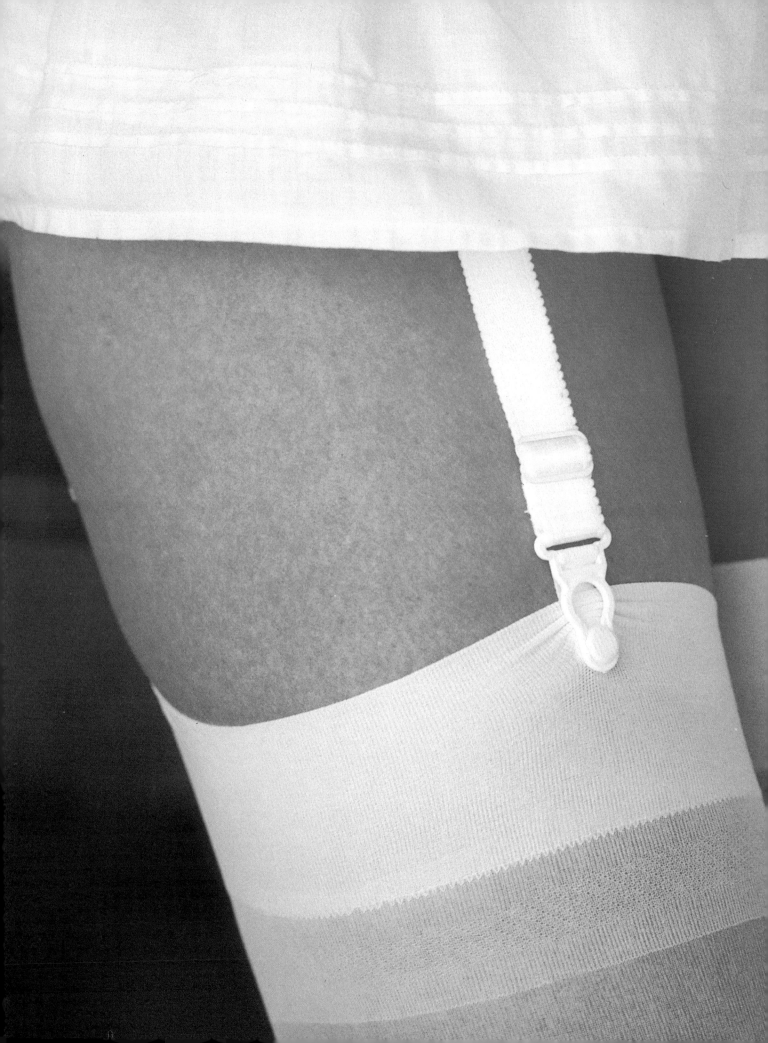

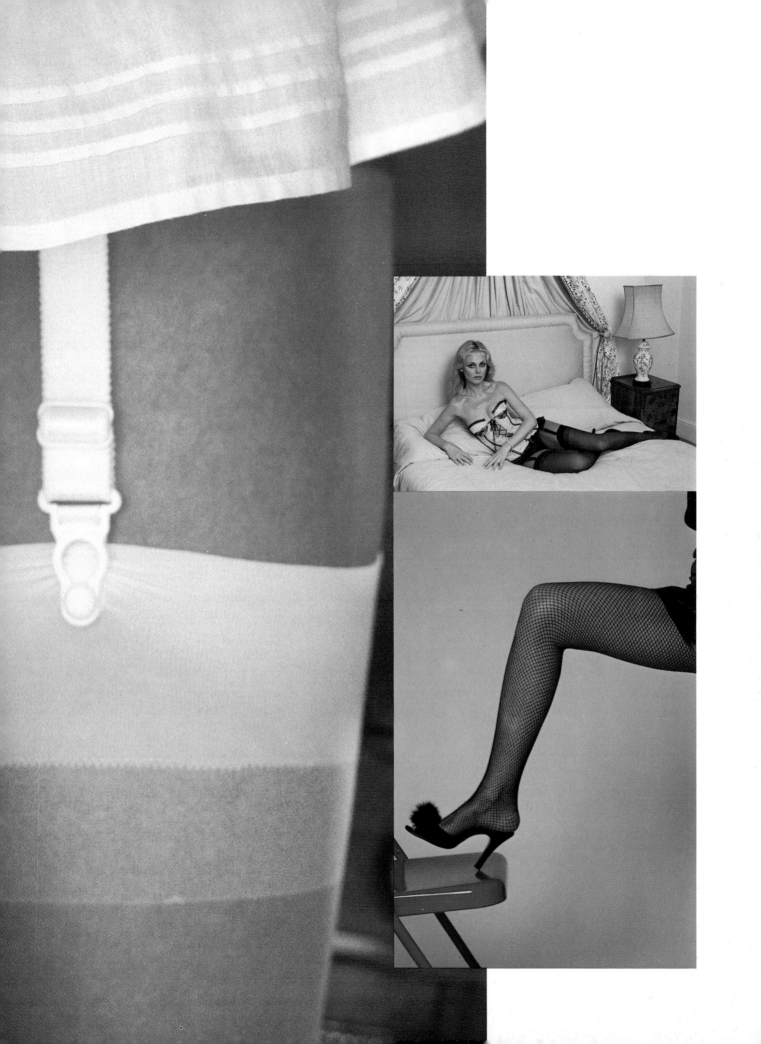

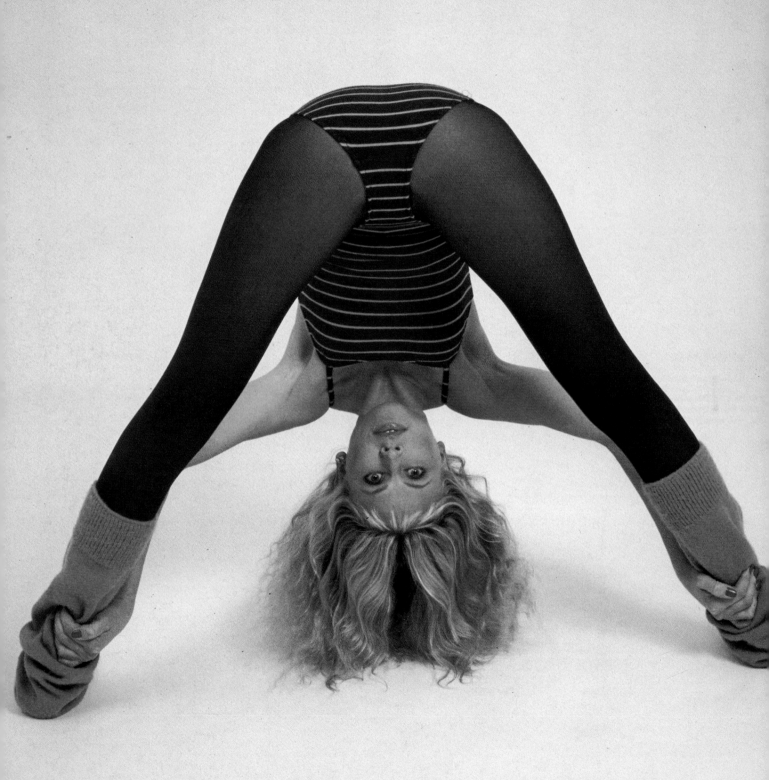

11/BODY TALK

Cats move sensually. We can learn a lot from their slow effortlessness, the way they take their time about everything including their morning stretch. Do you know how you move, how you look to others? Being totally aware of everything I do is part of my profession. In my early films looking at rushes wasn't to gloat over myself and my brilliant performance, but basically to see how I moved. Did I waddle like a duck, stick my bum out, or have my belly hanging over the top of my trousers? Or was my body held up straight as I sailed gracefully across the screen? The good part of all this self-awareness is that you carry it home with you.

Posture to Give You Confidence

No matter how beautiful you are, you can easily spoil it, so:

1. Don't stride or stomp across a room with hunched-up shoulders.

2. Don't waddle from side to side and look as though you have just parked your horse outside.

3. Don't have a cigarette dangling from your lips and drag on it in a fashion that would do Clint Eastwood justice. Not very feminine.

4. Don't twitch and twiddle and fiddle and 'can't sit still'. It doesn't matter whether you're tweaking the hem of your skirt or the strand of hair at the side of your face, it's nerve-racking to watch. I even had a girlfriend who pulled her eyelashes out one by one. How's that for signalling neurosis?

5. Don't slouch down on a sofa so that your double chins roll gently down towards your tum. Comfortable perhaps, but attractive never.

6. Don't sit hunched over if you've got big breasts, so that they end up near your tummy. Hunched shoulders are never elegant.

Bad posture is often the sign of someone trying to hide something – being too tall, or having too much bosom, for instance.

Alternatively it can result from some slight physical deformity. Flat feet, for instance, can give you a posture problem. I speak from experience and am highly uncomfortable in flat shoes as a result. Ex-fatties often hang on to their old posture habits and move ungracefully, partly because they hang on to their old image of themselves.

Poor posture is the cause of far more aches and pains than people realize. That nagging pain in your neck might not be from sleeping in a draught at all, but because you have one shoulder higher than the other. Your backache might be the result of having one hip fractionally higher than the other.

Stand in front of a mirror and let yourself go into your normal stance. See where you slouch. Turn sideways and do the same thing; you will soon see if your shoulders are hunched or your tummy is sticking out. Now draw yourself up to your full height, shoulders back, tummy in, and see what a difference it makes to your body.

I believe the best possible cure for bad habits is a good exercise teacher who will help line you up and tell you what to work on. She will tell you to think of yourself as a puppet with a string growing out of the crown of your head and running down your spine. Imagine someone giving the string a slight pull. It doesn't mean you should walk around with your nose in the air so everyone has to look up your nostrils, but just that your neck is extended and your head doesn't sink down into your shoulders. Your neck is not so likely to wrinkle that way, either.

Moving sensually has a lot to do with being confident. Don't wear clothes you are not comfortable in – a skirt that you feel is too short, a dress that's too tight. If you're self-conscious you can't be sensual. Avoid skirts that ride up and bra straps that keep slipping off your shoulder – fiddling isn't sensual. Nor is teetering around on too-high heels. The sexiest shoes in the world look ridiculous if you can't walk in them. Practise at home in front of a mirror before you go out in public.

If you are going to a party you will probably be holding a glass or a plate. If you're nervous, rather than trying to do a juggling act with your handbag you will manage better with an evening bag with a fine shoulder strap, to leave both hands free.

If you find yourself a temporary wallflower, you will look more approachable and less lost if you sip slowly on a drink. If you're left literally twiddling your thumbs, don't fidget, just clasp your hands lightly in front of you.

Don't be afraid to approach a stranger – remember, you are a stranger too. Asking questions is the best possible way to camouflage shyness and take attention away from yourself. If you are introduced to someone for the first time, extend your right hand in a firm handshake. Limp wrists aren't sensual.

Just as slow movements are infinitely more sensuous, so is leisurely speech. If you are nervous and blab away at great speed about nothing in particular, you will almost certainly scare people away rather than attracting them.

The most comfortable way to sit is to lean forward with your knees apart, especially if you are wearing trousers. Fortunately, wearing a skirt naturally encourages you to forget such ungainly habits. The prettiest way to sit is with your legs together and angled slightly to one side, not crossed at the knees because that restricts circulation. Smooth your skirt down behind you so that it doesn't get scrunched up while you sit. If you want to get cosy with someone, try sitting curled up in a semi-foetal position, which looks very feminine. Bodies do speak a whole language of their own. If you're perched on the very edge of your seat you'll look as though you're about to leave the room or feeling ill at ease. If you huddle in a corner of a sofa you'll look as though you're never going to leave.

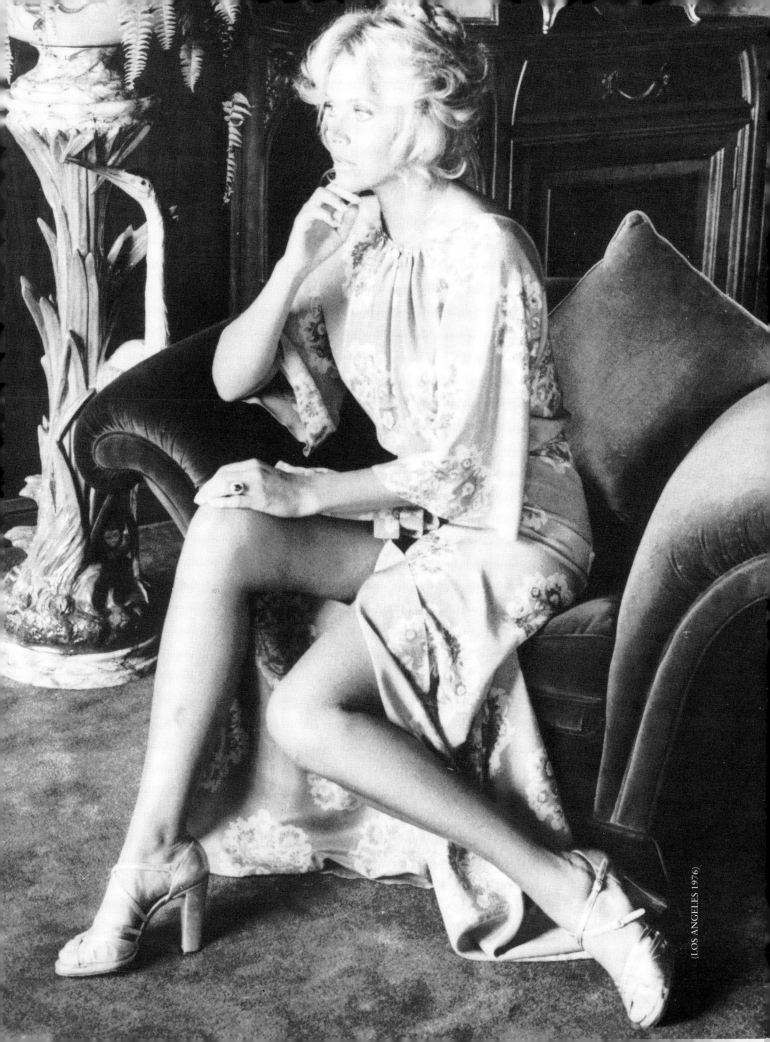

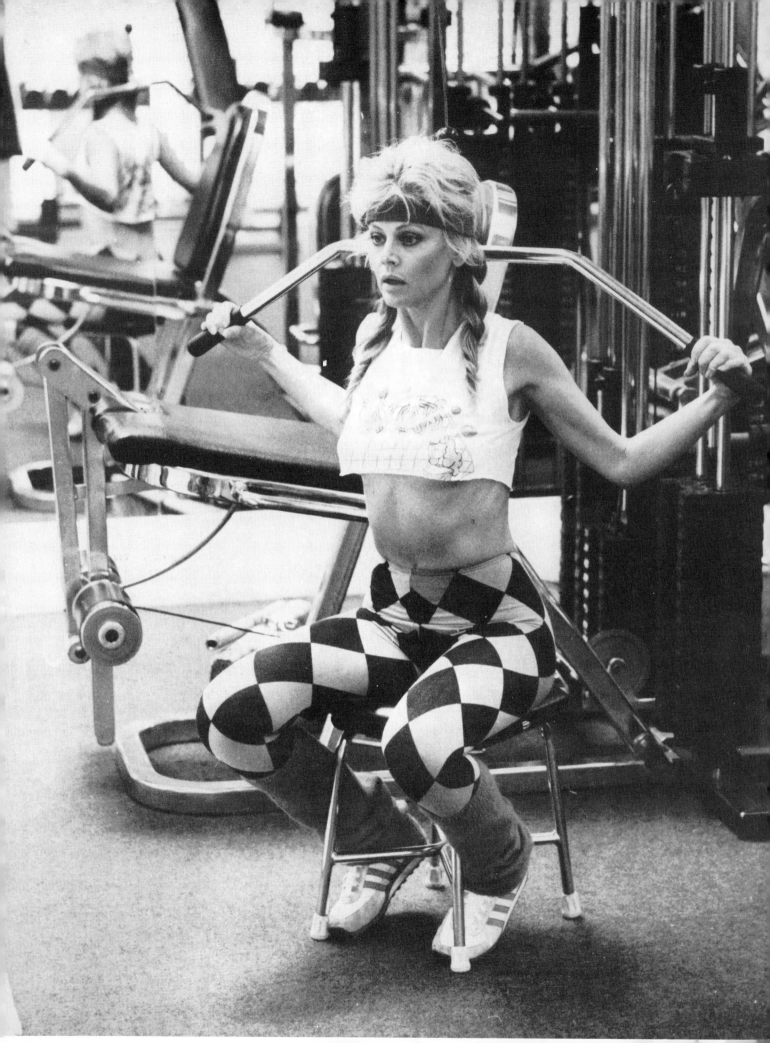

Shape up and Stay Trim

There's a camaraderie about exercise classes and I believe you need company. Although it comes down to just you and your body, and it's certainly not a competition, other people's energy feeds you and gets you going. There's no substitute for that. I don't suppose Princess Diana took her flopping tummy (it must have flopped at some point) to a class, but for the rest of us it's the answer.

If you want to develop your muscles you should take body-building classes. If you just want to tone them, stretching will achieve that.

Personally, I'm all for stretching and the point is to keep going further and further. You won't get your foot behind your ear on day one, especially if you're out of shape, but your body will amaze you with the progress it makes. As you get older your tired muscles tend to contract, and you're fighting a constant battle to keep them stretched out so you are fit and supple and firm.

Another terrific benefit of exercise classes is that even your face firms up. I've noticed that particularly since passing thirty. When I don't go to class my face seems to drop. Mind you, I don't believe in facial exercises as such. I think our facial muscles get plenty of exercise already.

Exercises are actually very sensuous, despite all the sweat and pain. Working in front of a mirror, confronting your own image, pushing your body, and subjecting your muscles to torture and doing it right, all feels very good. To me, apart from lovemaking and a couple of other activities, exercise is right up there. I really enjoy it. I'm in command and I'm pushing my body to the maximum. You've got to enjoy it otherwise you'll just make excuses and give up.

If you want to work out at home, try running up and down a little footstool, preferably backwards because that makes it tougher. That will get your heart beating. Take your pulse before you start and again five minutes later, and you will see the effect. Once again, you can't stop at five minutes but have to increase the duration each day.

I use a skipping rope and that's fun – it's good exercise because, like swimming, it uses arms, legs, stomach, the lot.

A trampoline is also perfect for streamlining your body. I bought myself a small one and jump up and down on it while I watch the news. It takes incentive, strength, and stamina to keep going. Five minutes will kill you at first, but if you persevere and work up to at least twenty minutes you will achieve as much as you would in an entire exercise class.

Looking Good While You Work Out

Don't think that just because you're going to sweat it doesn't matter what you look like. Give your body all the help you can by making it look as good as possible, then you will feel better about yourself. There are more don'ts than dos, but that's life!

1. Don't wear legwarmers pulled up to your thighs – they look like ice cream cones. Pull them down over your heel and just up to your calves.

2. Don't wear those shiny, one-piece leotards if you are overweight. If your bum is too big, wear sweat pants over your leotard or those lovely knee-length plastic exercise pants. They hide a multitude of sins.

3. Don't wear underwear under your tights.

4. Do wear a towelling headband. Regardless of trends they look pretty.

* Given the juxtaposition of bodies in exercise class and the spreadeagled positions one is required to take up, it should go without saying that exercise gear must get a good wash after each and every session.

Work out gear is important – the better you look the better you exercise

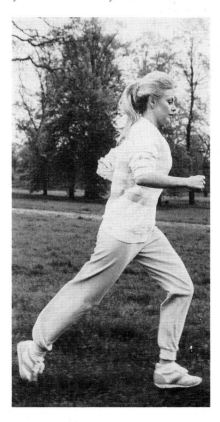

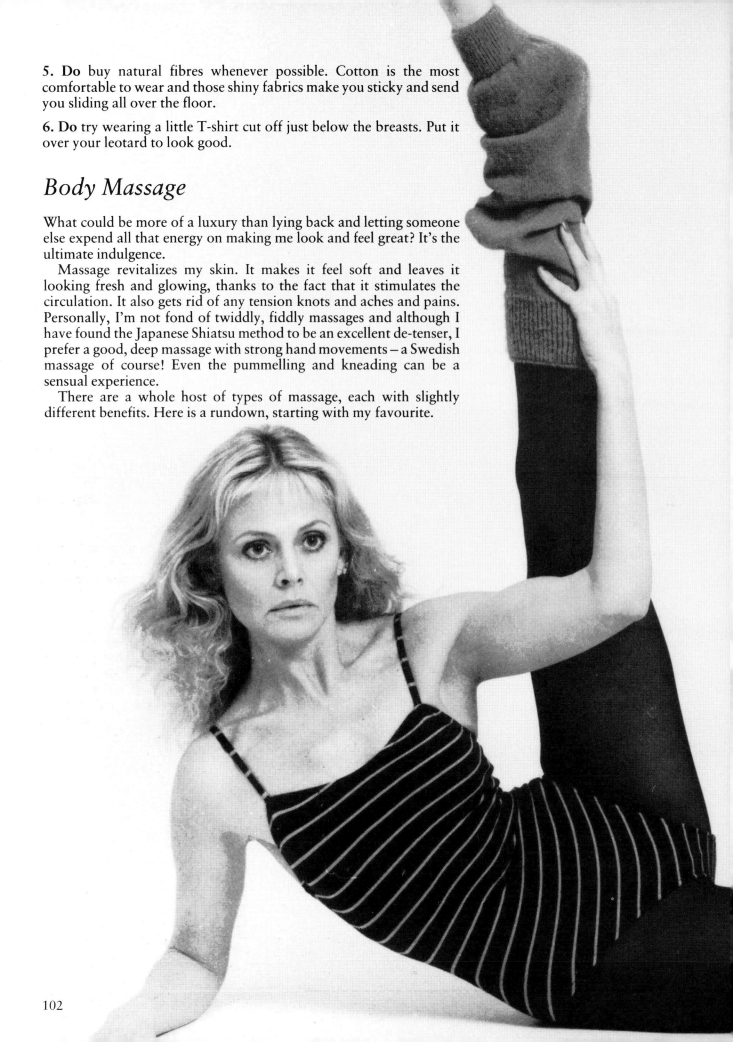

5. Do buy natural fibres whenever possible. Cotton is the most comfortable to wear and those shiny fabrics make you sticky and send you sliding all over the floor.

6. Do try wearing a little T-shirt cut off just below the breasts. Put it over your leotard to look good.

Body Massage

What could be more of a luxury than lying back and letting someone else expend all that energy on making me look and feel great? It's the ultimate indulgence.

Massage revitalizes my skin. It makes it feel soft and leaves it looking fresh and glowing, thanks to the fact that it stimulates the circulation. It also gets rid of any tension knots and aches and pains. Personally, I'm not fond of twiddly, fiddly massages and although I have found the Japanese Shiatsu method to be an excellent de-tenser, I prefer a good, deep massage with strong hand movements – a Swedish massage of course! Even the pummelling and kneading can be a sensual experience.

There are a whole host of types of massage, each with slightly different benefits. Here is a rundown, starting with my favourite.

Swedish massage is the most widely available and is often used by back specialists and physiotherapists because it can help relieve fibrositis and muscle and back problems. This method starts with slow stroking and builds up to kneading, pummelling, tapping and slapping. To my mind it's just the thing if you're tired and aching.

Shiatsu is an ancient Japanese method, a near relative of acupuncture. The massage puts deep pressure on acupuncture points and nerve endings and is worth a try if you have sinus or headache problems or find yourself under a lot of stress.

Aromatherapy is a bit like a combination of the first two, but its prime distinction is the use of pure plant oils massaged in for their healing properties. It's probably the most sensual of massages because the plant aromas are so wonderfully soothing. Aromatherapists claim that each of the oils has different properties – for instance, camomile calms the body and mind.

Connective Tissue Massage tackles flab and fat. The fingertips and knuckles are used in a fairly fierce fashion to break up fatty deposits. You can have a go at this yourself in the shower on your hips, bum and thighs. Always use upward movements – massage strokes should always be directed towards your heart.

Reflexology is based on the belief that there are reflex points all over our feet which are terminals for all the different parts of the body. Pains in the feet are used to interpret problems elsewhere. The actual foot massage is deep and energizing; afterwards you feel as if you are floating on air.

You don't have to hire an expert to make use of some of the benefits of massage. Once you've experienced a few professional treatments it's certainly possible to adopt a few of the simpler movements for home use.

Body creams and lotions work far more efficiently if you massage them in rather than just smoothing them on to the surface of your skin. I use deep, stroking movements, all directed towards the heart.

You can make a whole romantic ritual out of heating up some massage oil and massaging your mate by candlelight with soft music playing in the background. I know people who use mutual massage as a seductive prelude to lovemaking, but I'm not much for that sort of thing myself and neither is the man in my life. I can give a good, strong massage, but I don't do it for sexual purposes – I'll do it for someone who has hurt their shoulder or leg or has a tension headache. I must have a good touch, because once I start people can't get enough.

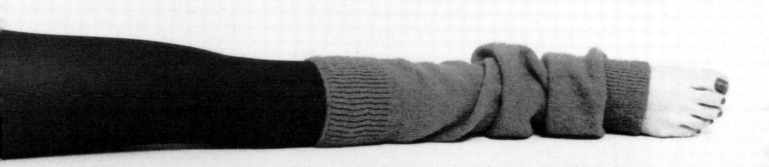

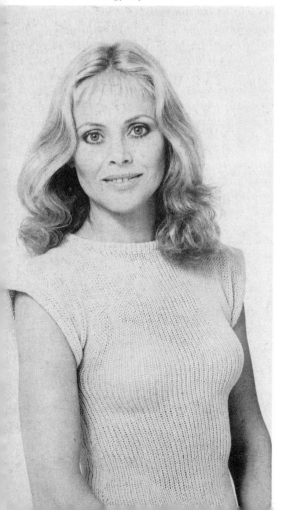

*Even a small bust benefits from a bra
under a clingy top*

Underwear can make or break the way you look in an outfit. The most sensual silk jersey dress can be ruined by bra hooks and a pantie line peeping through, not to mention the lumps and bulges caused by too tight undies.

Underwear should enhance your best points while minimizing your figure faults. It takes time and patience to find the one bra that fits perfectly, the one style of panties that are comfortable and flattering, and the one brand of tights with just the right leg length. When you *do* find them I'd buy five of each and resist the temptation to stray towards something that catches your fancy in a shop window but that you probably won't wear. I have drawers full of underwear I never use, so I speak from experience. Underwear can be pretty, or sexy, but it should always be comfortable.

The Bra Debate

I am very much in favour of bras for any woman who needs support. While I don't believe that going bra-less causes your boobs to fall to the floor – although that may be partly true for someone endowed with more than 36 inches – neither do I believe in letting big breasts bounce around all over the place. I don't think it looks good and I imagine it's very uncomfortable.

I don't wear bras that often – frankly I don't need to. My breasts are on the small side and I still live under the illusion that my bust looks OK without a bra. Until I catch a glimpse of myself that changes my mind, I shall continue.

Men don't seem to mind small breasts. Whenever I've broached the subject of having implants, there has been an outcry. Besides, implants don't look altogether natural. They might be great in clothes, but when you lie on your back they defy gravity and point skywards, they don't fall to the sides like the real thing, and they are so firm you can hang things on them – so I'm told by women who have them.

I don't wear bras under silk blouses because I think it's quite attractive to see a bit of nipple through the silk. Even if the nipple is a bit low, it doesn't matter.

It *does* matter under tight, clingy T-shirts or jersey dresses or wool sweaters, and then I think small-breasted women, myself included, should wear a bra. Although with exercise you can keep your bust pretty much in the same place, there's no doubt that age and having

COND SKIN

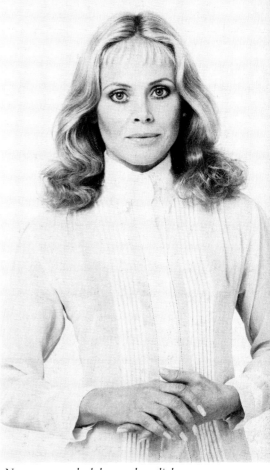

children will take its toll. Besides, some clothes simply don't flatter breasts without the help of a bra – sweaters especially. That's why I tend to wear a bra much more in England or elsewhere in Europe because then I'm wearing my cold-weather clothes.

Sometimes it's a question of modesty. While I think that it can be quite attractive to expose a little nipple, if for instance you have a job you have to decide how much you want to expose and be prepared to take the consequences, to suffer or enjoy the stares and sniggers and glances. While I never wear a bra around the house I often put one on when I'm going out to meet people. Sometimes it's just more comfortable to know that my breasts are under control some place slightly above their natural position.

There are lots of pretty half-cup, underwired bras but since they are invariably uncomfortable I'd reserve those strictly for occasions when you're planning to undress in front of someone. For everyday I'd go for a fairly sheer, fairly natural-shaped, full-cup bra with a bit of support.

Never wear a dark bra under a light-coloured blouse, and if you've got the right figure, you won't need a bra at all

Buy black to wear with black and flesh colour to wear with everything else. Pretty though white is, if you are working it is impossible to keep it snowy white. A white bra is something I'd keep for special summer days and holidays only.

Bear in mind, when you buy, that lace looks pretty but it should be smooth or it will show through your clothes. The same goes for fastenings – make sure they lie flat to give a clean line. Always try the bra on and check the back as well as the front. Make sure the elastic isn't too tight at the sides or back – if it cuts into your flesh it will lead to bulges. Make sure the cups are the right size – lean forward and let your breasts fall naturally into the cup to check.

However pretty it looks, don't buy the kind of bra that consists of one elastic band around the back and one over each shoulder and comes in a package with a pair of panties. They make you look exactly as you did without a bra, if not worse. They have a knack of making breasts point downwards in a highly unattractive fashion.

If you are really on the small side, I'd buy a nicely padded bra. There are moderately padded and extremely padded bras, depending on the effect you want.

Before buying any bra, I'd suggest putting your shirt or sweater back on and making sure that you like the look it gives you.

If you're full-breasted you should always wear a good, firm support bra under your exercise clothing. Buy one specially since, in this instance, the wider the elastic the better.

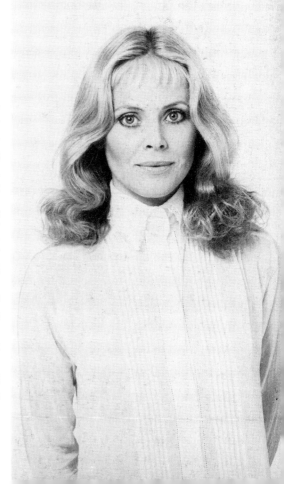

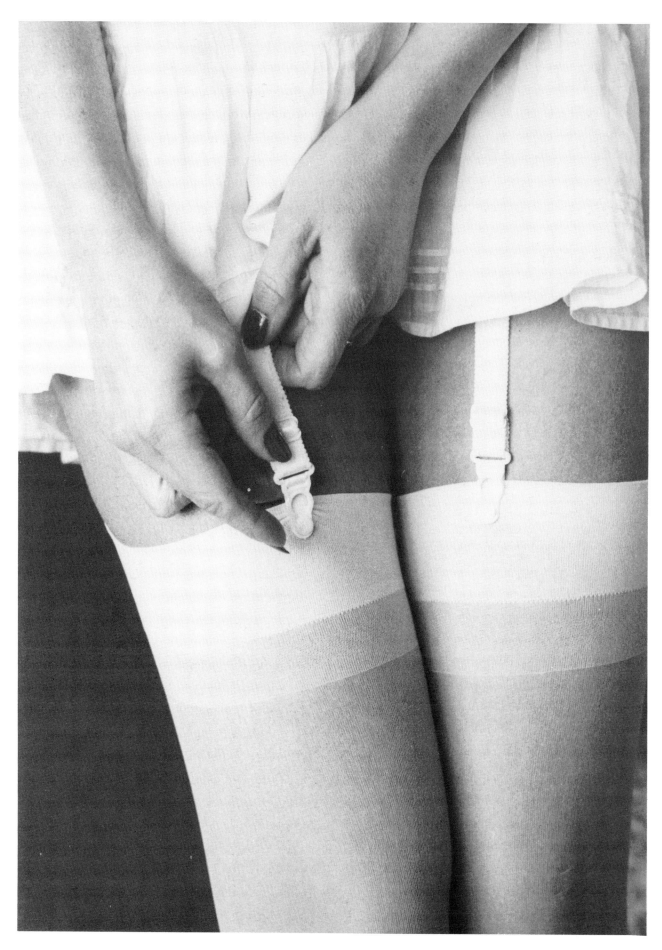

Panties

To me these are an alternative to tights, and I'd never wear both. The object of tights is to get a nice smooth line, whether it's under an evening dress, a daytime dress, tight trousers or jeans. Plonking on a pair of panties too simply defeats the purpose. But make sure your tights have a cotton gusset.

In a warm climate like California one rarely wears tights or stockings, so panties are a must. Whatever your build, for everyday wear comfort is the top priority. If that means they're bikini-brief or come all the way up to the waist, so be it. Once you've found a style that looks good under your skirts and trousers, stick with it.

I have two kinds that work well for me. One is a tiny triangular shape with little spaghetti straps at the sides, but you have to be reasonably slim to wear it. Under very tight-fitting or clinging clothes I wear a strange-looking item which has no back, just a front, and looks much like a G-string. Since it doesn't cover your bum you do need quite a good shape to carry it off, particularly under a clinging dress. Under jeans it doesn't matter as much since the fabric is firmer.

Cotton and cotton-mixture panties are your best bet in a hot climate. Wear nylon by all means, but only if the crotch is reinforced with cotton. Never wear anything nylon directly next to your delicate female parts or you are asking for a yeast infection. Cotton breathes better and helps body sweat dry faster.

I've bought my favourite panties in beige, red, black, every colour under the sun. It's fun to match your bra if you are wearing one, but the most versatile colour is flesh – that way you don't have to worry about what you wear on top. There's nothing worse than seeing blue and green patterned panties peeping through pale trousers. The front may look fine but the bum's always a giveaway. I can't understand any woman going out without checking her rear view.

Like bras, panties should be a perfect fit. If they are too tight they'll cause ridges and spoil the smooth line of your clothes.

Vests

They make a good extra layer under winter woollies. I wear them because I don't like the feeling of wool next to my skin, but that's purely personal. Thin cotton vests are best, with thin spaghetti straps. Buy a size too small so that it isn't lumpy under your clothes, spoiling their smooth lines, and doesn't add volume.

Suspender Belts

These aren't exactly a commonplace item in the 1980s. They're not terribly practical, unfortunately. To make them look their best you put your panties on first, then the suspender belt. But how do you go to the loo? If you put the panties on top you lose the prettiness, but you can't have it both ways.

Suspender belts are fun for special occasions, though. Let your man feel a little bit of suspender during the course of the evening and he'll go crazy, I guarantee it.

Either match your undies or your stockings. Black silk stockings are, naturally, very sensual. They're expensive but worth it. Seamed stockings are also very sexy – sandal-foot style, of course.

Slips

Worn under skirts and dresses they can eliminate a lot of wrinkling. I'd choose a full-length style an inch or two shorter than my skirt length. The plainer the better, so it doesn't add bulk. Even fancy lace can create ridges under a thin top. I'd avoid pure nylon and ask for anti-static, cling-free fabric. Black is fine under dark clothing, but again you'll find a flesh colour the most versatile buy.

Tights

For the best visual effect they should be totally sheer from top to bottom. I can't bear seeing myself in those matronly pantyhose that are reinforced from the waist to the tops of the thighs, and I certainly wouldn't want my man to witness such a spectacle.

If you are a touch lumpy and bumpy and want to look a fraction thinner, I recommend slightly stretch control tights. Elbeo and Givenchy make them. They're more expensive but they really are good and suck everything in.

---

* If you are wearing tights with no panties and are worried about a little leakage, wear a panty shield. They're shaped like a sanitary towel but wafer thin and so tiny they're barely visible when they're in place. You peel a strip off the back, rather like a sticking plaster, and they stay in position perfectly.

For everyday wear in the office or at home, I'd buy one-size-fits-all, nothing fancy. But always buy the kind with a sheer foot, which are so much prettier than the reinforced ones.

If you get a run while you're out, there's always the old nail polish trick – colourless, of course. I once went to a disco in a very short black dress and very sheer black tights with diamanté designs on them. Suddenly I noticed a huge run all the way up my leg. Since I don't wear panties underneath, my remedy was to slip into the bathroom and cut the legs off, leaving myself wearing the pantie part. Thankfully my legs were tanned at the time!

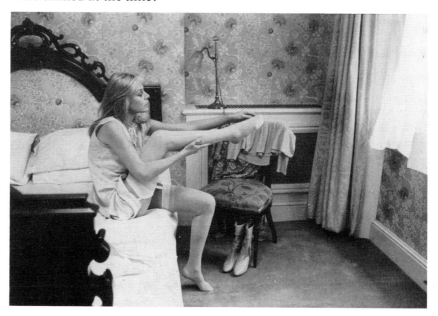

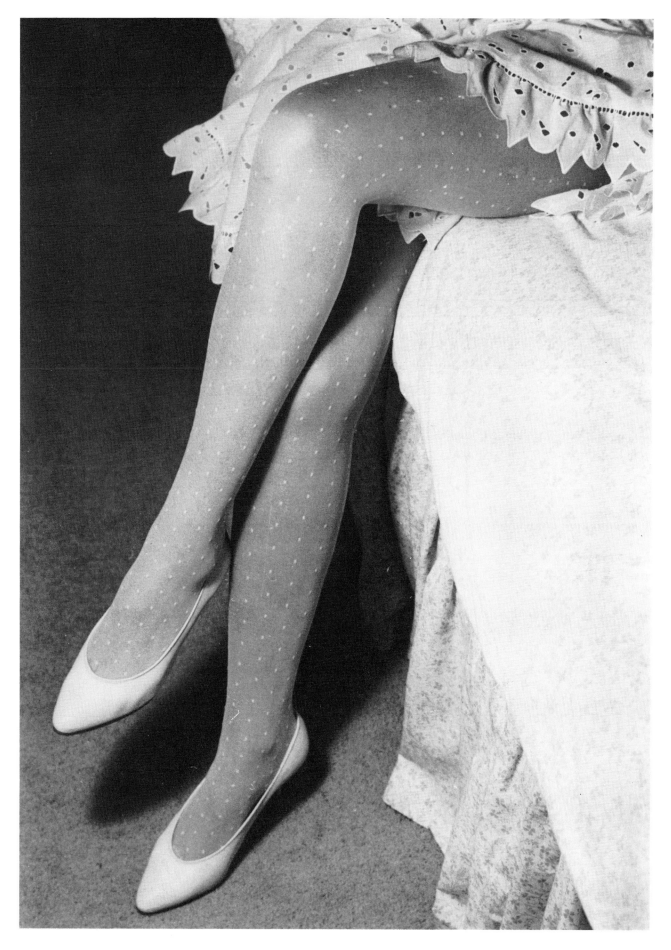

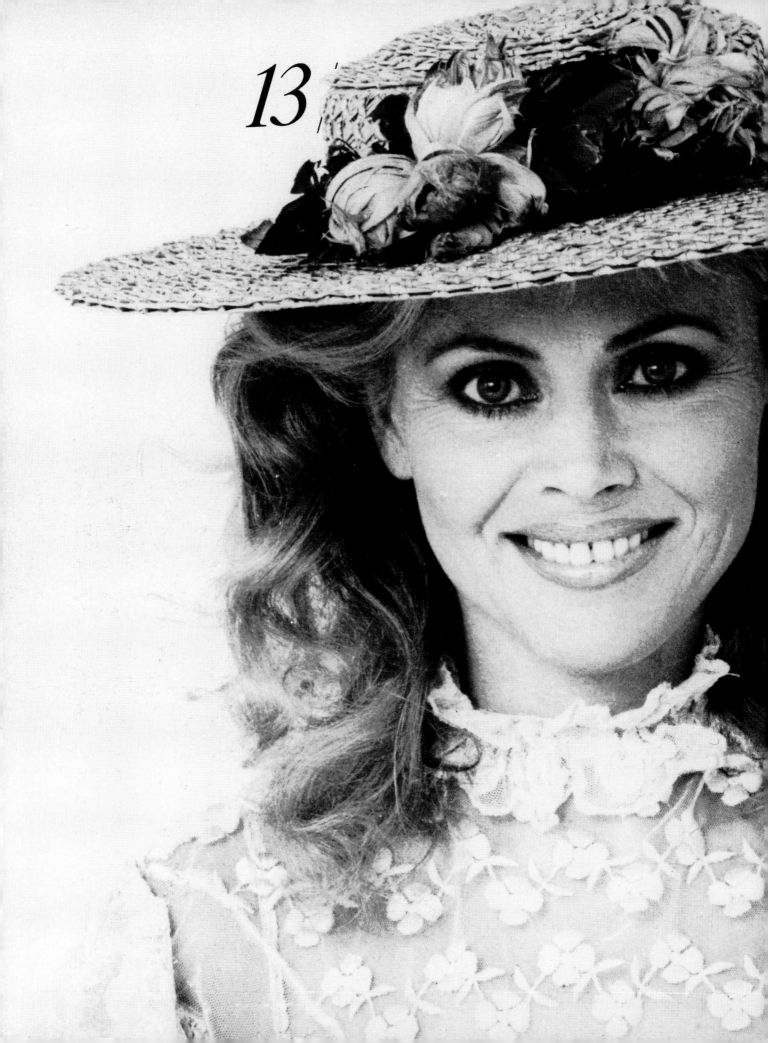

13

LOTHES: PUTTING THE ICING ON THE CAKE

I dress for no man, I dress for Britt Ekland. I can wear a black leather motorcycle jacket one minute and a ladylike suit the next, a rockabilly outfit or a fabulous, full-length silver fox, but my style is always indisputably my own. It wasn't always so.

When I was twenty-one I looked fifteen and was married to a man twenty years older than me, whom I desperately wanted to complement. All my married life I dressed ultra-conservatively in the well-cut little Wallis copy of the Chanel suit, the Knightsbridge horsey-set black and white organdie-collared dresses, the mink coat and the crocodile bag. I look back now at photographs taken twenty years ago and see someone far more mature and sophisticated-looking than I am today.

I felt much more liberated after my divorce, but obviously if you live with someone you have to make concessions. Today everything I put on makes me feel good about myself, and that's the key to sensual dressing.

Touch is important – I love sumptuous suedes, silks, and furs, and believe they are well worth saving up for. Slinky satins are also sexy. Anything that feels rich is sensual.

I put a lot of money into rubbish when I was young, buying incredibly expensive clothing like sequinned disco suits which have absolutely no value today. As I got wiser and more mature I started buying things that I am proud to say have today increased in value. I won't spend £100 on a dress I'll wear once. I can't. I made mistakes but I won't make them again. Most of the things I've bought through the years I can in all honesty say I can still wear today.

Clothes can be a solid investment. I don't particularly like the word 'quality', but quality does pay. I have sequinned 1930s' evening gowns for which I paid less than £250 apiece in the antique market. Today it would be more like £1000.

Appreciating just as fast are my antique fans and bags. They are so beautiful that I hang them on the walls so that I can enjoy them every day, like pieces of art.

It's lovely to be given jewellery, but the advantage of buying it yourself is that you get what you want. When I was twenty-one, Sellers gave me a diamond-studded watch and a triple-banded Victorian ring. Fortunately, he did have good taste. Way back in the 1960s he bought me my first gold Rolex and I in turn bought him the man-size one. Mine was stolen in 1972 and I couldn't afford to replace it until I went to Hong Kong in 1976. In 1978 I treated myself to the diamond bezel and diamond face that they introduced. It's now worth twice what it cost. Not a bad buy, eh?

My main philosophy is, if you don't truly love something, don't buy it. When you look at something and your mouth literally waters, then get it even if it means scrimping and saving.

It's taken a long time to get to this point, but today *we* make fashion – fashion doesn't make us. Dressing has to be an individual choice and is mainly a combination of what suits you and purely personal taste.

If you want proof of everlasting love, I have the only designer gown my mother ever owned. It's a Balmain, a thick satin dress that she bought in the 1950s which now suits me perfectly.

I've had other long-term love affairs. I bought several of Zandra Rhodes's original dresses back in the days before she had any factories, and the Zandra Rhodes Lou Adler gave me for a birthday ten years ago was a green fur jacket with pink insets. I still wear it and love it. If you can't afford designer originals, search the second-hand shops and antique stores. The stuff is all out there if you take the time to look.

Even trouser suits can be bought to last. Five years later you may have to change the width of the trousers but that's it. A blazer's a blazer's a blazer, whether it's 1940s style with big shoulder pads and large lapels or narrow-lapelled with a single button. Some things just never go out of fashion.

Dream Buys for Sensualists

If you live in a cold climate, why not dream of having an incredible sable coat? You can always settle for a coyote. That's a beautiful blonde fur and very reasonably priced.

If you like fur, wear it. If you feel guilty about it, don't. I have a 1920s' leopard-skin coat and I don't feel bad about wearing it. It's older than I am! I don't like my dogs lying on top of me, but I do like the feeling of fur. There is something very glamorous about it and definitely sensual. Certain animals are bred for their fur like mink and chinchilla, just as certain animals are bred for food like Aberdeen Angus bulls.

Only movie stars and pop stars can afford floor-length furs. If you can't afford a below-the-knee fur, rather than save up for that silly wrap that aristocratic folk wear, I'd buy something else. I don't think jackets are worth the investment unless you've got masses of other coats in your wardrobe, in which case fine, buy a white fox jacket or white fox stole.

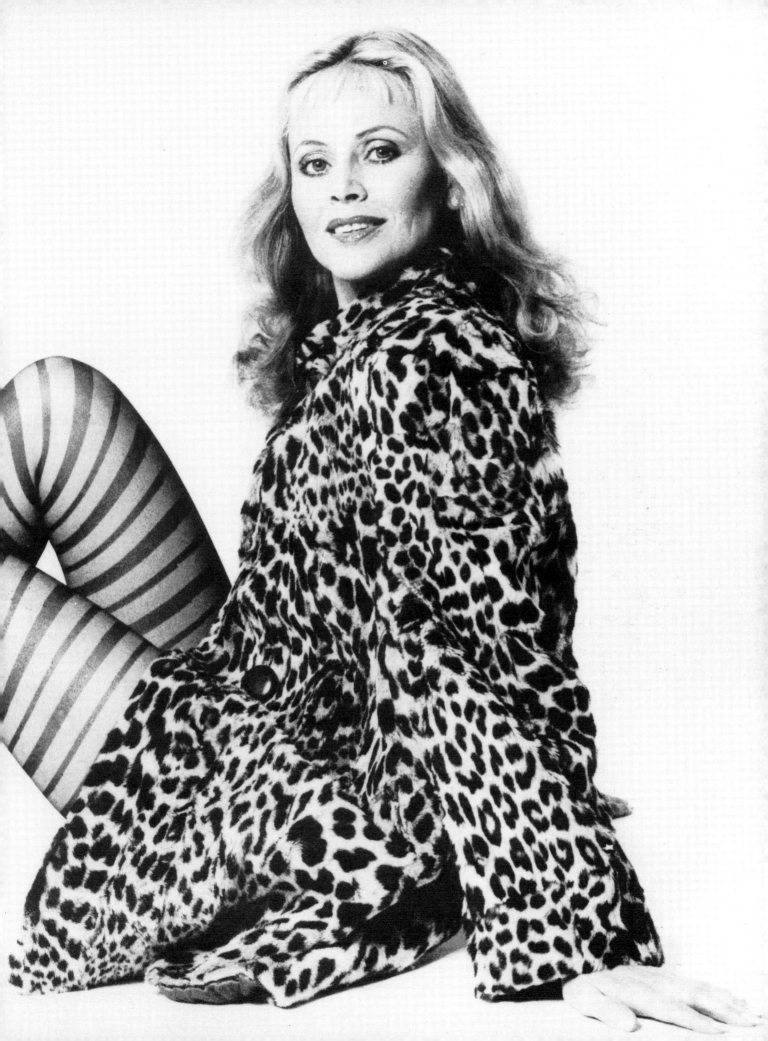

Fur-lined cloth coats look good, as do some cheap furs dyed in pretty, fun colours. If you can't afford the real thing I wouldn't bother – I don't see the point in fake furs.

My next dream buy would definitely be a good suede outfit because suede looks so expensive. Of course it *is* expensive and a trouser suit might set you back £250, but it's worth it. Suede today is beautifully soft and silky and you can wear it day or night, summer and winter. It's not seasonal like wool or gabardine. Providing you don't buy something ultra-trendy with batwings and tails hanging off it, it's something you can wear for the rest of your life and it won't wear out.

There's nothing I love more than wearing my punky, short, black leather mini-skirt with fishnet stockings and high heels, but that's a fad. It's sexy and it's spur of the moment, so you can't plan your wardrobe around it. But suede you can, every time. I'd go for a jacket and trousers that you can wear together or separately. You can wear the jacket with another pair of trousers or the trousers with a big sweater. Tan is a good all-time colour.

Silk shirts are classics. Everyone loves and wants a white silk shirt because they look and feel so good, but admittedly it's expensive and it has to be dry cleaned. The practical alternative of course is black. I'd go for both if you can afford it – a white, man's-type silk shirt and a black, mandarin-collared, plain shirt. I have black silk Yves St Laurent shirts with mandarin collars from 1964, and no one's any the wiser because the collar is so classic. I'd buy a black velvet silk ribbon or a black chiffon scarf and wear it as a tie on the white shirt. That looks sexy.

When you buy silk shirts make sure you are wearing the bra you will wear under it and that the shirt doesn't gape at the front or pull across the back. If the armholes are too tight when you try to embrace someone, don't buy it.

If you buy a shirt too small you will also perspire like mad and it shows very quickly on silk. If you perspire a lot, it's worth buying dress shields and just tacking them into the armholes of your shirt to protect the fabric. It only takes a few seconds and for an expensive shirt it's worth the trouble.

If you have a reasonably slim figure, I would definitely buy a white suit, but not linen, even though I love it, because it wrinkles too much. You only have to breathe to put creases in it. I'd go for white gabardine or very light wool, very plain, nothing high-fashion. Personally I'd buy a jacket and trousers and if they have a skirt to match buy that too – then you're literally set for every occasion. You can wear the white jacket with a black shirt, black skirt or trousers, or with purple or pink or blue. Or the other way round – put a silk shirt and belt with the trousers or skirt. The permutations are endless.

Basic Buys

Classic slacks are a good buy that you will still be able to wear in five years' time. White, beige, black, grey, or red go well with silk shirts. If you are slim I'd go for plain, well-fitted ones to show off your figure – dead straight legs and side pockets. If you're very large yet you insist on wearing trousers I'd choose a style with pleating across the front, fairly loose in the leg and not too tight across the bum or tum. To my mind the most flattering look of all for larger ladies is a fairly narrow-leg

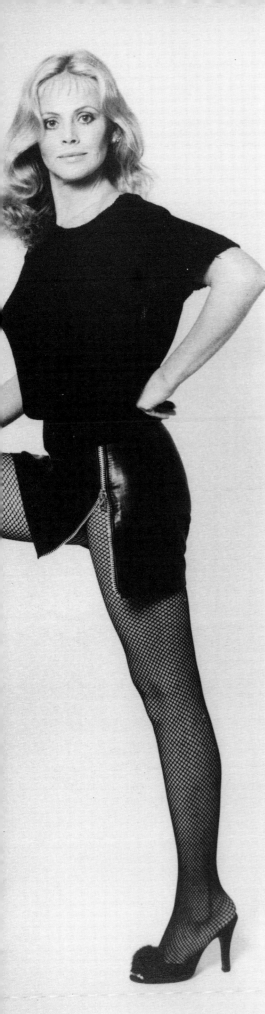

trouser with a tunic over it. It looks very sexy to wear thin crêpe trousers and a big flowing shirt top with high heels.

If you haven't got much money, don't forget that different-colour accessories (see pp.121-5) can create a completely new outfit. Rather than rushing out to buy a cheap dress just so that you have something different to wear, I'd wear the same dress three nights in a row and just change the shoes, the earrings and the hairdo. Ninety-nine times out of a hundred, I guarantee your man won't even notice.

Jumpsuits are useful garments to wear around the house. They're not terribly sensual – unless they are silk – and are not for anyone to take off other than yourself. Nor are they wildly practical when it comes to going to the loo, particularly in winter when you have to do a striptease and sit and shiver. But, and it's a big but, they are incredibly comfortable and I do believe it is important to have one set of comfortable clothes. It could be a jumpsuit, or it could be sweatpants and a sweatshirt, or a big man's shirt and a pair of patched jeans. Whatever it is, you should feel very much at home in it.

You shouldn't always feel the need to be on show twenty-four hours a day. Once you have become a sensual woman you're sensual whether you're wearing jeans or black satin.

I'm not crazy about T-shirts although I love freebies. I don't like wearing anything initialled or carrying other people's advertising, unless it's for The Stray Cats, of course! The only exception I'd make would be for Levi jeans, and that's because they're virtually a tradition now that they've been around so long.

Jeans are something I'd treat with caution. Unless you're the shape of a model your rear end never looks that good. There are lots of clothes more flattering than the average blue jeans. The only pair I wear are my beau's and he has a much slimmer figure than me so I have to be careful, otherwise I look overstuffed. They're too long, but since we share them I have to compromise and roll them up.

Each year I'd say it's fine to spend £100 or so, according to your means, on some fun clothes that you know will just see you through the summer. I bought a pair of pink suede court shoes for £15 and I love the way they look with a pink summer dress right now. Next year it will be something different, so it's not worth spending more.

I realize that few people can afford to buy *Vogue* and *Harpers and Queen* every month, but even if you buy a copy just twice a year you will get a pretty good idea of what is in fashion. Some of the looks are so extreme that even I wouldn't wear them, but some are very good and it's revitalizing to get that input. It can make you look at your wardrobe in a new way.

Figure Faults and How to Hide Them

I know all the tricks of the trade. If I am overweight no one knows unless they see me with my clothes off. When I was pregnant with Nicholai I wasn't married to his father, Lou Adler. I felt there was a certain stigma attached to being an unmarried mother so I didn't want anyone to know.

I immediately adopted the layered look – tunic tops over longer skirts with Victorian petticoats peeping out from under the skirts. I would top that with yet another layer – a long-line, flowing jacket. I wore long, trailing, floaty scarves to camouflage my tum.

Thankfully today's fashion freedom is helpful. No one is forced to wear mini-skirts or clumpy, club-footed shoes. Nor does anyone have to wear those dreadful dirndl skirts with multitudinous gathers round the belly which make you look like a walking lampshade. Here are some figure disguise tips:

If You Are Overweight. . .
1. Shoulder padding works well – nothing extreme like a David Bowie or Flash Gordon costume, just gentle padding so that your shoulders are at least as wide as your hips.

2. Always wear dark colours below the waist and light above. If you do it the other way round you will be literally highlighting bulges.

3. Always wear vertical stripes everywhere, top and bottom, no matter what the persuasive saleslady says. Better still avoid stripes altogether. The heavier you are, the less you should wear patterns.

4. Blouson tops are very flattering. You can even wear a straight skirt underneath since the blouson style hides your middle.

If You've Got a Very Broad Bum. . .
1. A straight-line shift dress or a bias-cut skirt or a straight skirt with a tunic top over it will all work wonders.

2. Forget whether it's in fashion or not, always make sure that your shoulders are wider than your posterior, even if it means living with shoulder pads for the rest of your life.

3. Try never to wear trousers. If you must, stick to the kind that Greta Garbo or Katharine Hepburn wore in the 1930s – gabardine slacks with wide legs, parallel from top to bottom. Never wear narrow-bottom trousers if you're broad in the beam; they will only accentuate your problem.

4. Don't wear standard-fitting T-shirts or very clingy tops. Avoid all narrow tops. In summer why not wear an oversized T-shirt? If you want to make it looser and fun-looking, cut off the neck ribbing. There's nothing to say you can't wear fun clothes just because you're big.

5. In winter you can wear long tunics all the way down to your knees if you want. Mandarin collars look good. Find a nice, straight dress that you can cut short to wear over trousers.

6. If you are short, suffer and wear high heels.

If You've Got Fat Arms. . .
1. Cover them up, even in summer – gauzy fabrics do the trick without making you melt.

2. Don't buy shoulder-strappy, waisted things because the fat at the side of your breasts just pours out and the fat at the back will peep over.

3. Batwing sleeves are also pretty because they are narrow at the wrist, yet hide a multitude of sins around the shoulders and upper arms.

If You've Got Good Legs, but Not Much Else. . .
No matter what current fashion says, wear short skirts, beautiful (seamed) stockings and high heels. Just show off your legs and cover the rest. I have friends with plump middles who never wear leggy clothes, then suddenly one day you discover they've been hiding the most gorgeous pair of legs. What a waste!

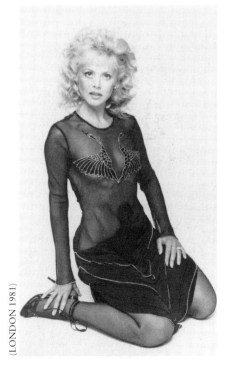

(LONDON 1981)

116

If You've Got a Good Bust and the Rest of You Is Lousy. . .

Wear full-length, low-cut dresses. Do what Joan Collins does and show off your bosom whenever you get the chance.

If You're Small and Thin on Top but Your Legs Aren't Terrific. . .

1. Wear waisted things with tight, fitted middles and show off your best point.

2. Wear bare, strappy tops.

Evening Glamour

Dressing Up

If you are going to have one evening dress and one only, I'd say your best buy is a slinky, black number with spaghetti straps. If you've got a pretty good figure, then buy a fairly fitted style. If you haven't, it could be waisted with a flared skirt. If you've got bad upper arms, go for a ruffly, off-the-shoulder shape where the ruffle disguises them.

Black dresses are infinitely versatile. You can wear them with last summer's white silk jacket or an embroidered jacket or a sequinned, antique jacket. You can accessorize with gold or midnight blue.

Alternatively, a deep burgundy red velvet dress is useful if you live in a cool climate, and if you go to a lot of black tie parties you will need a change.

If you look good in blue, midnight blue satin is very dramatic and looks pretty shimmering under the lights. It could be low-cut with spaghetti straps or tight-bodiced with a removable white organza collar and a fullish skirt.

Don't feel obliged to match your shoes and stockings to your dress. With midnight blue, for instance, pink shoes and stockings look pretty, red shoes and stockings look dramatic, shimmering silver looks glamorous. The combinations are endless and you needn't be conventional as long as your shoes and stockings match.

If you like the Victorian look, all laced-up and white and virginal, that's a good look for evenings, too. If you have a tan that you want to show off, you can't beat a white, slinky, classic, strapless or spaghetti-strap gown. Why not have a slit skirt? Slits at the sides or back or front are very sexy and sensual as long as you don't show your panties or tights. If you've got good legs, make the most of them. High-heeled sandals are a must.

Sensual fabrics for evening are silks and satins – even synthetics – lace and chiffon and crêpe. Body-clinging bias-cuts are sexy if you've got the figure for them.

If you're past forty and your body isn't in good shape, don't pretend that your arms aren't overweight and that the rolls of fat don't hang over the back. Go for the Marlene Dietrich trick instead. Wear a gown with a gauze overlay or a low-cut dress with chiffon insets or a sheer overjacket in lace or chiffon or crêpe. Wear a dress with a high-neck lace inset to disguise a scrawny neck. Keep up the mystery. A batwing-sleeve blouson style in black crêpe can also hide that which is not fit to be seen.

Once you've got your perfect evening gown, don't spoil it by having it the wrong length. It should just touch the point where your shoe heel starts. If it's longer, it will be virtually impossible to move. Don't have a hem because you can catch your heel and trip and break every bone in your body.

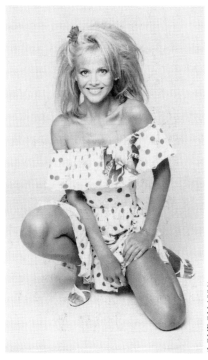

(LONDON 1981)

117

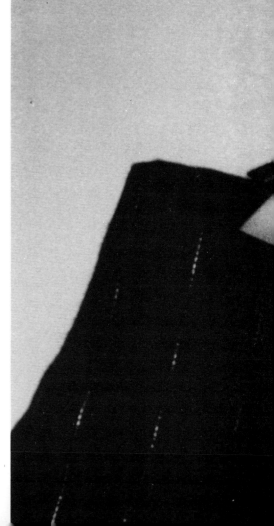

For a smart coordinated look, a hat and gloves can pull it all together

Covering Up

Bare-shouldered dresses are all very well, but unless you're getting door-to-door chauffeur service you could freeze to death while you scour the streets for a taxi.

Princess Diana is forever stepping out of limousines into the cold winter air, but at least the royal cars are heated. For those of us whose skin is bluer than our blood, capes are an excellent invention. Velvet always looks good and if you are the adventurous type you could even make one yourself. The bias-cut kind are no more complicated than a circular tablecloth with a hole in it; otherwise look round second-hand clothes stores or antique markets.

The beauty of capes is that you can even put a cardigan under them and no one will be any the wiser. Whatever you do, avoid a knee-length coat or fur with a long evening dress sprouting out underneath it. Either wear a short fur jacket – you can hire them quite reasonably for the evening – or have a short dress. It's a shame to go to all the trouble of choosing and buying and wearing a beautiful dress and accessorizing it right down to the satin shoes, only to ruin the entire effect with a reversible mac.

Hats Off

I happen to look good in them, but overall I consider hats strictly non-sensual. I can't understand why any woman insists on wearing one of those woolly tea-cosies with a bit of fluff around the edge. The only thing marginally worse is a pair of fluffy ear muffs. Hats are functional items in cold climates, and that's about it.

One exception I sometimes make is to wear antique beaded skullcaps. You can pin them on to the back of your hair and they look very pretty. If you want to wear a false hairpiece and don't have time to fiddle with it, a skullcap covers a multitude of sins.

Hats can be very inconvenient. They invariably fall off when a man kisses you, or they blow away in a breeze and get run over by cars. Those little twenties' pillbox hats with veils look mysterious, but are highly annoying when you forget you are wearing them and want to get something out of your eye.

Hats do look good on Princess Diana, but who can afford her milliner? Unless you're *sure* they really suit you, I'd get a cheap straw hat for the holidays but that's it.

118

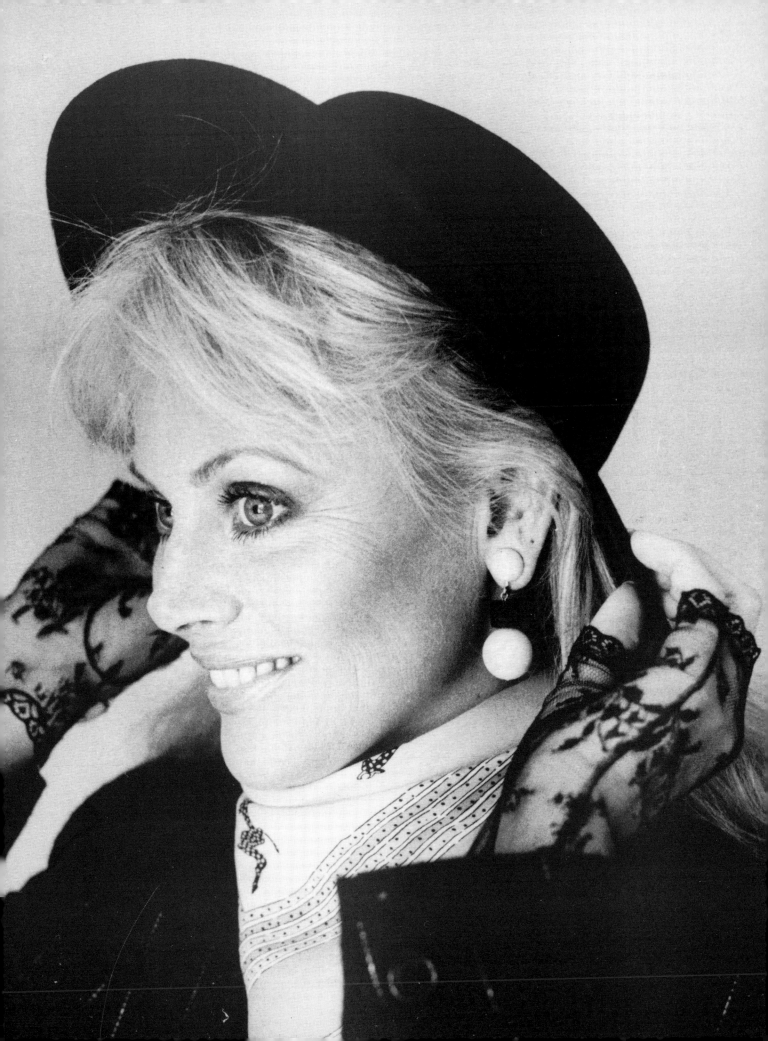

Shoes Are My Passion

I think I must have walked in every type of shoe ever made during my lifetime. Those platform-soled, treetrunk-heeled monstrosities of the seventies must have been the most outrageously ugly look of all time. Looking back I can't believe I wore them, but I did. Here are my tips on how to make and keep a perfect shoe collection that will, I hope, stop you making some expensive mistakes and contribute to the overall impression of you as a sensual woman.

1. Everyone should own one pair of very practical, very plain, basic pump or court shoes with a very high heel. They never look wrong.

2. Want to walk sensual? The best bet for evenings at home are high-heeled slip-ons (mules). High heels every time. I personally have flat feet and wouldn't be seen dead barefoot, not even in a film. High heels are a must. To put the whole sensual look together, match maybe a champagne-coloured satin robe with champagne-coloured slip-ons.

3. The easiest classic shoe to wear at night, summer or winter, is the open-toed, open-heeled style with just one plain strap across the front. The strap should be not less than one inch wide and preferably closer to two inches.

4. I know you have been seduced by those little spaghetti-strap shoes that look unbelievable, but you will have the most miserable time of your life wearing them because no stockings or tights or strong feet on this earth can stop the straps cutting straight into your flesh.

5. The same goes for those Roman sandals which the saleslady spends ten minutes winding up your leg. Of course they look gorgeous because you have your foot in her lap. Forget standing up in them. Either you look as though someone has tried to strangle your leg or the whole thing falls off. There is no happy medium.

6. Ankle straps are an infinitely safer bet because you can always punch another hole in the strap. Wear the straps as loose as you comfortably can, though, because if the ankle strap cuts into your leg it has a nasty habit of making it look like the end of a sausage.

7. Everyone should indulge themselves in one pair of splendidly expensive evening shoes – really superb classics in just plain suede or plain satin. I wouldn't go for open toes or sling-backs and I wouldn't go for white because what can you wear white with in winter? You can dress up the basic shoe by clipping on a pair of incredible earrings or shoe clips, or you can make your own pompoms from feathers and pin them on.

8. Buy a pair of high-heeled boots. The difference they can make under a pair of jeans is unbelievable. Someone who looks like a little, squat dumpling in sneakers will suddenly grow tall and long-legged. I know it is incredibly impractical to suggest high heels for walking through the snowy, wintry streets of Stockholm or New York or London. Trying to negotiate snow with ice underneath is lethal, I know. So go for boots with a wedge heel and non-slip soles. They still give you a bit of a lift and unless you are Twiggy with two sticks that you can literally stuff into anything, that is what you need.

9. Wedge sandals never go out of style. You can't go to the beach in heels, and wedges look better than flats.

10. **Don't** wear open-heel shoes with either tights or stockings that have reinforced heels and toes. That really makes me cringe.

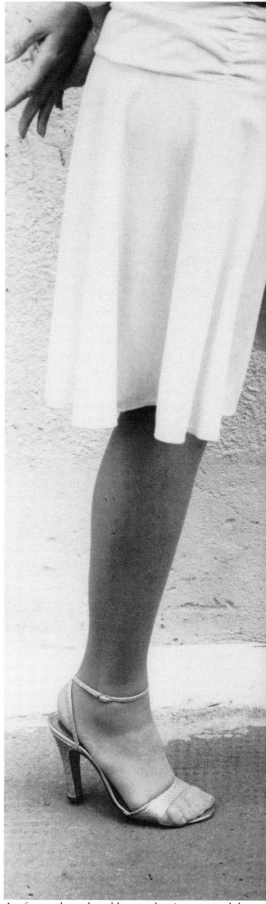

I refuse to be seduced by spaghetti-strap sandals,

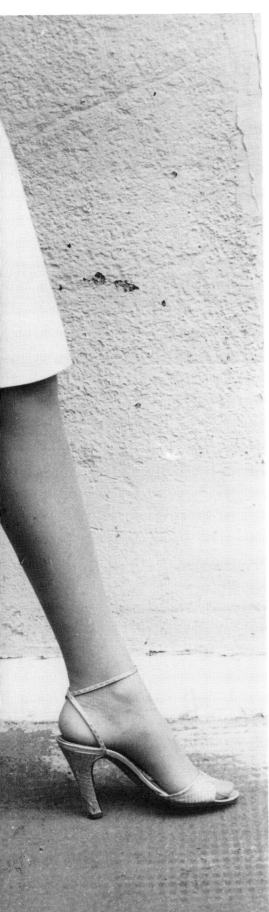

but ankle straps are practical and *pretty*

11. **Do** remember, when you buy, that all mature women swell to a certain extent in their legs and feet. Allow for it.

12. **Don't** wear white shoes with tan stockings. That look is strictly 1959.

13. **Don't** wear shoes that are so uncomfortable you have to slip them off under the restaurant table. It always makes me laugh when you see a really elegant woman in diamonds and coiffeurd hair, the lot, and there under the scalloped tablecloth she has got her shoes off.

14. **Do** take care of shoes. Nothing looks uglier than scuffed heels, and decent shoes deserve a bit of love. One day a month I make sure all mine are immaculate. I polish leather and brush suede with a suede brush. If I drive in high heels I keep a towel in the car and slip it over the rubber mat to protect them.

15. **Don't** wear good shoes in the kitchen or bathroom. Not only will you ruin the flooring with high heels, but there is a good chance you will spill toothpaste or cream or talc on your shoes. Just try getting talc out of black shoes when you're already running late. I always tell Victoria not to wear her suede boots in the kitchen but she claims she's just making a salad or something. Well, one piece of lettuce with salad dressing is all it takes to make a nasty greasy mark on them.

16. **Do** stuff shoes or boots with newspaper if you don't have shoe trees. Boots should always be kept standing upright with a rolled-up newspaper inside so they don't bag out of shape.

17. **Do** pack shoes and boots in individual bags – just plain plastic ones will do. It keeps them from scuffing.

Colour Guide
I love black shoes above all else. They're highly sexy and very good-looking. Red shoes can also be very sexy as long as they're not patent. Stick to suede or satin or plain leather. Red patent leather looks fifties and cheap.

If you'd like a light colour, go for natural tan which blends with your leg and makes it look longer. It goes with red, blue, green, purple – anything. Tan shoes make your legs look as though they've just grown out of the ground. The foot doesn't become the focal point so much – you just notice incredibly long legs. To me, that coming-from-nowhere look is the sexiest and most sensual of all.

Shoes in the Bedroom
Pretty shoes should be the last thing to come off – there's definitely something sensual about stripping with high heels on. Obviously the same does not apply to your hiking boots – that's in the same league as a naked man in black socks. But high heels are very flattering when you are getting undressed.

Don't wear boots that require a man's muscle to remove them. There's nothing attractive about your hanging on to the bedpost while he puffs and pants and the damn things won't budge.

Sensual Accessories

Shawls for Feeling Feminine
I have the most amazing fringed red cashmere shawl. It's so huge I can wrap my entire body in it. I won't mention the price because it would

feed a family of four for two weeks, but it's so fabulous and so sensual that I consider it worth the money.

If you can't afford cashmere make sure you choose something soft. Lambswool or even a wool and synthetic mixture can feel good. Whatever it looks like I'd put it round my bare neck and feel it before buying, to make sure it isn't itchy against my skin.

Of course red cashmere or wool aren't right for summer, but I wear it indoors or outdoors in the autumn. It looks great over a white silk blouse, red skirt and boots, or with a red polo-neck, red beret and matching cashmere mittens. Just for show I'd wear my silver fox coat with a red beret, red polo-neck and gloves with my great red shawl on top, but that's really signalling 'Please notice me' – that's being Britt Ekland.

Apart from being eye-catching it's actually a very practical extra layer or cover-up. If I could buy just one shawl I'd maybe opt for a colour other than red. Red's sometimes tough to wear if you live in a cold, blue-nose climate. I'd choose black or beige or light tan, all of which go with almost anything.

Summer shawls are a great cover-up, especially on holiday. I like the westernized version of the kind of wrap you see men and women wearing in India and Thailand. Buy a large square of good-quality cotton, patterned or plain, and hem it round the edges. Use it to wrap round you at bust level to cover a bikini, not to mention the lunch you've just had in your bikini. As long as it's totally square you can fold it diagonally and use it as an evening wrap – the finer the cotton the better. Something with a gold or silver thread through it looks effective with a tan. Make sure the fabric is soft, though. If you've been sunning yourself and your skin is sensitive the last thing you want is something scratchy wrapped round you.

Scarves were once a passion of mine. If you look at old photos of pop stars and movie stars, including yours truly, you will see a multitude of them. I used to wear the long, floaty kind when I was pregnant with Nicholai to disguise the bulge. Although they've since doubled as headbands and belts, I don't find much use for them today.

I do use scarves to tie up my hair but silk, however sensual, doesn't work on hair because it slips right off. Slightly crêped fabrics are best, like cheesecloth and crinkly cottons. Coloured cotton squares work well, too. Don't overlook antique and second-hand stores as a source – some of the fifties' designs are great fun, especially those with people on them and dogs and cows.

Bagging It

I used to have a large collection of handbags but unless they're the soft, crumply kind that you can roll into a ball, how do you travel with them?

I have good Gucci crocodile bags in every colour you can imagine but I swear I haven't touched them for fifteen years. Somehow I've come full circle to the point where I was in my teens with pairs of shoes – one brown, one black.

I'd choose leather or suede for bags every time. I hate vinyls unless it's the kind of fun design that shouts, 'Hi! I'm a vinyl bag.' Never buy anything that pretends to be something it's not, and that includes leather stamped with an alligator skin imprint. Even though it's leather, it's not alligator and someone is bound to spot it's a fake. What's the point?

If you live in Europe, particularly in a cool climate, the best all-purpose buy is a medium-size shoulder bag big enough to hold your make-up bag, cheque-book, comb and purse. Buy not too pale tan or

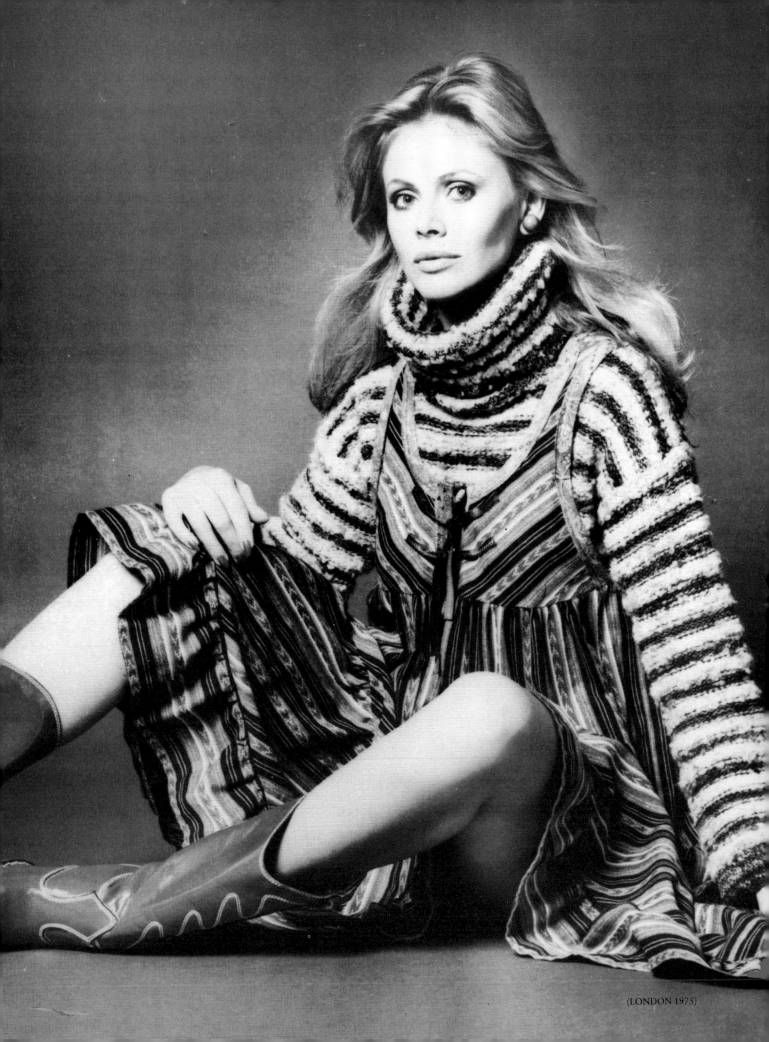

(LONDON 1975)

basic brown suede or leather. The saddle-bag style with a flip-over top is always stylish with a winter coat and boots or even with a fur. Ideally I'd buy one brown, one black, to go with nearly all my winter clothes, but greens go well with brown, burgundy with black, and so on.

When I'm in California I have a different bag philosophy. The distances are so vast that I can start out at 10 a.m. and not be home – three meetings and an exercise class later – till ten at night. Unless I want to turn my car into a semi-trailer, my solution is to have a large, pouchy shoulder bag and keep a small clutch bag inside it.

The large bag houses everything from a big diary to exercise clothes to my make-up kit and even a script or business papers. If I'm meeting someone for lunch, say, and I don't want to take the big bag with me, I just pull out the clutch bag, pop in my lipstick and money, put the big bag under the seat, and lock the car. (Burglars take note if they want to pinch anything from me!) I stick to the same basic colours, black, tan, or brown, in leather or suede.

In summer, of course, you can buy pretty, light, cheap clutch bags to your heart's content and they look good matching the colours of your summer clothes. I'd also buy a nice shoulder basket or a canvas bag with leather reinforcements and strap, for when there's a bit more to carry.

For evenings, you can't go wrong with a perfectly plain black bag in either silk, artificial silk or silk moiré – either a clutch style or one with a shoulder strap. Beyond that you can pin on an antique diamanté pin or any other pin you fancy and that will make it look like a million dollars. In summer, for a change, get the same bag in white.

A clutch bag always looks very elegant at night, although I personally tend to favour shoulder bags because they're easier. I like having my hands free, but it's a matter of taste.

Belting Up

If I could afford it I have no doubt that I would buy everything Barry Kieselstein-Cord ever made. He's a New York artist who, apart from amazing jewellery also makes belt buckles and tips in silver or gold, all signed and incredibly stylish. The belts are often lizard and once you've got the basic buckle and tip you can buy every colour you care for from pink to purple, from turquoise to peach. They come in all widths, depending on how rich you are. I have a very thin one. Brown's in South Molton Street, London, sell them – failing that, you can always buy copies.

Luckily, belts are the one thing you can really go fake with, and if you find a cheap style that you like I'd buy it in as many colours as you can afford.

Right now I have a lot of belts with metal studs – I like that heavy-metal look. It's fun to wear more than one belt at a time, but you've got to be thin to do it. Wear a slim one around your waist and a wider one below. For summer it's fun to play around with ropes and hessian. Try mixing a rope with a silk scarf – just twist them around together. If you are feeling creative, make your own very special belt by buying an Art Deco-type buckle and sewing it on coloured elastic or velvet ribbon.

When you buy belts make sure that they fit into the belt loops on your trousers without twisting. Mind you, a very narrow belt looks equally silly in very wide loops. It's best to wear the particular outfit when you try the belt on in the shop.

The same goes for skirts, if they have belt loops. Even if they don't, I think a slim belt adds the finishing touch to a skirt and shirt.

Belts can be a good disguise – for a waistband held together by a safety pin, for instance. They're also a clever way of hitching up a dress into a blouson tunic, or of shortening a skirt.

Never belt thick clothes such as sweaters, coats, fur jackets, quilted fabrics because it will make you look too bulky. Avoid wearing two belted things at once – pants and jacket, for instance. It looks too messy.

Avoid belts that are too long. I hate it when the end hangs in mid-air like a strange tentacle. Use double-sided tape to keep it in place or, if you know you're going to stay the same weight, have it cut to length. Get a good shoe repairer to do it by taking the excess from the buckle end, which is neater than dealing with the problem at the other end.

If the belt is very, very long but very slim, try tucking the end under and tying it into a loose knot. That can look quite effective.

If you need to make an extra hole – if it's a man's belt, for instance – make holes all the way along, spacing them evenly. It looks smarter. Punch holes from the back and then from the front so that they are smooth.

Hand Signals

Gloves were the rule of etiquette when I was growing up in Sweden. They were also a necessity. They save your hands in both a dry, hot climate and a very cold one and I like them. In my time I've been known to buy twenty pairs of white leather gloves although I admit that's rather excessive.

Suede or leather gloves are infinitely more sensual than woolly, knitted ones, although I'd make an exception for cashmere. Fur-lined gloves are cosy if it's very cold. If you can't wear leather and have to wear wool I'd go for mittens, they keep your fingers warmer. Leather gloves are best for driving since they don't slip on the steering-wheel.

To me gloves are a fashion item. I have a collection of original hand-crocheted cotton gloves, pretty see-through ones in white, pink, purple and blue, to wear with my Victorian petticoats and lacy tops.

If there is an occasion that calls for a black suit, I like to team it with a white hat and white gloves. If you can afford it, invest in a white pair, a red pair, and a black pair, preferably in soft, fine leather.

Let's say you've got a black dress, incredible red shoes, but you feel there is something missing. You don't have a red handbag, though you've got red lipstick – red gloves will pull the outfit together. If you don't want to spend the entire evening wearing gloves, take one off and put it in your handbag. One glove is a nice affected look and of course you wear all your jewellery on the other hand!

In summer I'd buy a selection of pretty coloured cotton gloves. They're inexpensive and they can really round off an outfit. You could literally wear the same dress all week, one day pink accessories, the next day purple, the next day blue. Since you don't have to pay the earth for them, why not?

I'm not keen on long gloves. You can't really wear rings or jewellery with them, whereas short gloves look pretty with a watch or bracelets. If the gloves are a bit on the long side, push them down on your wrist, rather like those boots that rumple softly around the ankles.

If you've stopped smoking or biting your nails, gloves can be a godsend to stop you twiddling and twitching.

14 / JEWELLERY: A GIRL'S BEST FRIEND

Jewellery can feel sensual, but only to the wearer. I somehow don't think the feeling of a diamond-studded hand, a chained neck or a diamond-dripping ear is a particularly sensual experience from a man's point of view.

Pearls are the only kind of jewellery I believe you can call sensual, and I am passionate about them. I think they are more becoming on a mature woman than on a young one, but they have a beautiful sheen. Sellers told me at a very tender and impressionable age that pearls are for tears, so I'd never owned a pearl in my life until Christmas 1982 when my friend Billy Gaff gave me a fantastic seven-stranded pearl bracelet. Pearls are the only comfortable jewellery because they are totally smooth and rounded, with no hard edges. Cabochon-cut stones, which are rounded rather than sharp-edged, can also be very sensual.

Women always study me. I can plug in and hear them whisper, 'Are those diamonds real?', 'I wonder where she got that?' I can hear them thinking out loud when I'm all dolled up in my best bits.

American women still tend to favour great big mountains topped with a variety of stones. I find that sort of jewellery very cumbersome and ageing. Jewellery should not just prove your wealth — that's playing games.

Buy Real

I know you can buy great fakes for £100, but you'd be better advised to take that £100 as a down payment on something real. You will feel better about what you are wearing, feel better inside yourself, and wear it with more pride.

Good jewellery is an investment. I'm not saying you are going to double your money when you sell, but you can usually count on getting your money back if you buy wisely. Quality is important — anyone can buy a diamond, but there is no guarantee it's a good diamond so try and get impartial, expert advice.

If you are buying for yourself, decide what you would like to collect and stick with it. If you like diamonds, then go with diamonds.

Your first investment should be a pair of diamond stud earrings. You can wear them in bed, at the office party, to the beach, everywhere. Unless you cover your entire face with hair, stud earrings are the most noticeable.

Right and following page: I love classic diamond or gold jewellery – you can't go wrong with the real thing

126

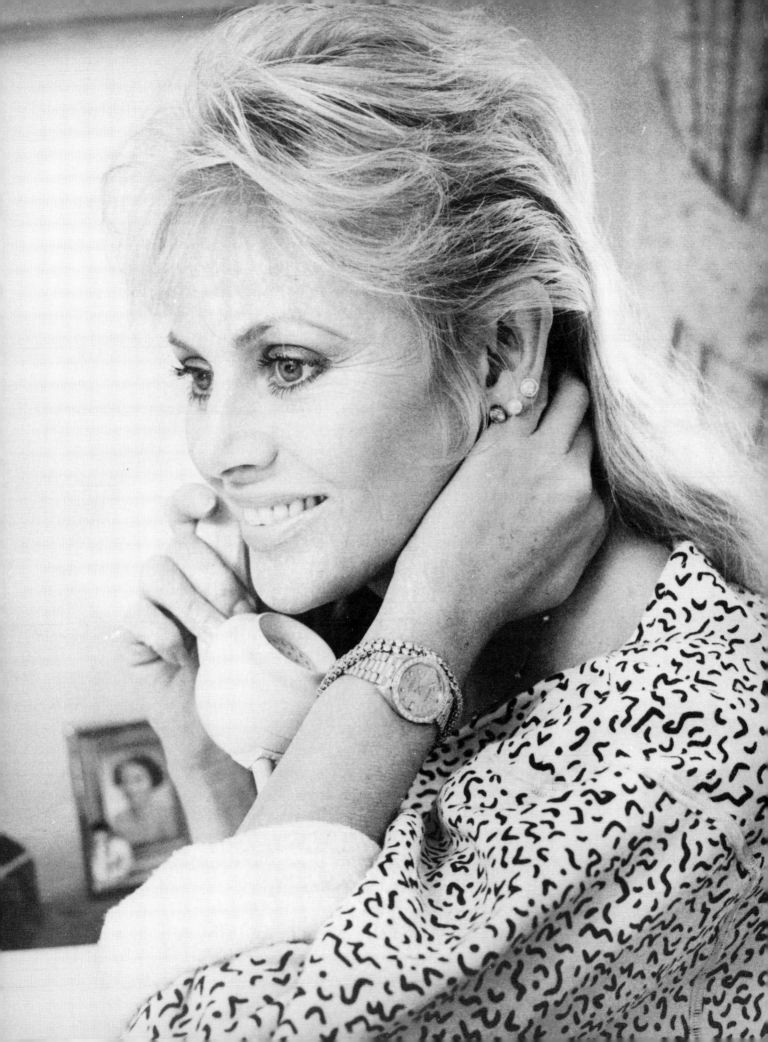

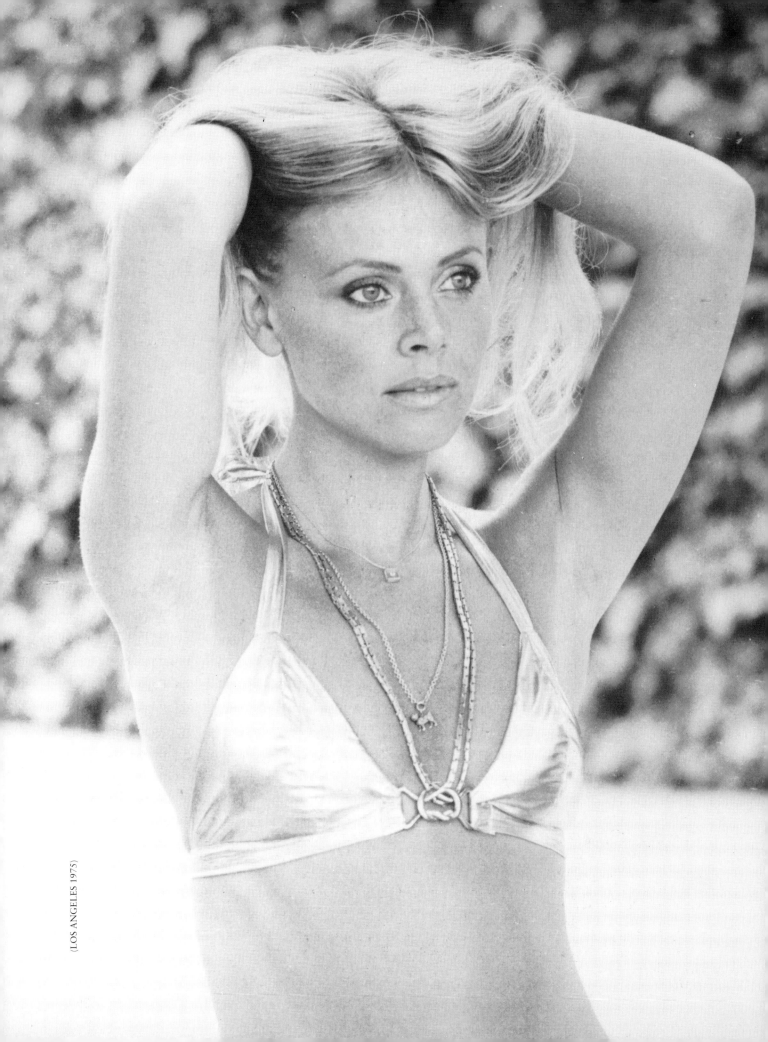

I bought a single-stone diamond ring for investment purposes, but since that always has connotations of love and romance it's not much fun to buy it for yourself. Instead I would go for a diamond heart on a thin chain – the heart should sit neatly in the 'V' of your throat. You can wear it with absolutely everything except polo-necks.

I'd rather see a pretty little chain around a less than pretty neck than nothing at all. Better to focus on that than on an expanse of scrawny neck, in my opinion.

If you want the bare look, but you know that your neck's not great, you can always cover up with a high-neck dress and a bare, bare back. You can wear brooches and pins on the front of the dress, though not a necklace.

Day for Night

Time was when we discriminated between daytime jewellery and night-time jewellery. I don't believe in categorizing it like that. If it makes you happy and it looks good, wear it.

I wear my antique Cartier watch surrounded with diamonds and jet with black leather jeans and a black leather jacket in the middle of the day. Why not? I wear my gold Rolex any time of day or night. I would wear my two very fine diamond bracelets (one set in white gold, one in yellow) without blinking with blue jeans and ostrich boots and a tailored suit jacket.

There is one exception I make, based purely on taste. I have an incredible white gold and diamond watch with a very flashy coral face, but it looks too obviously an evening item to wear during the day.

Stay in Style

If you wear gold, wear gold. If you wear silver, wear silver. Don't mix the two. If you want to wear big, sparkly, multi-coloured, multi-stone extravaganza rings and purple plastic hanging butterfly earrings, go ahead. Why not add that heavy gold-looking chain with the big mounted coin as well as all those mock turtle plastic bracelets?

If you are going to look like a Christmas tree, go with it all the way. Or else go classic, and stay simple and uncluttered with neat diamonds.

Consider colour, too. Don't mix jade with a ruby, or topaz with a sapphire. The colours are too much together. It's best not to mix precious with semi-precious stones in fact, unless you want to put an opal or turquoise with diamonds; diamonds are subtle enough not to clash with anything.

Keep It Clean and Safe

There is nothing sadder than seeing a beautiful diamond earring clogged up with shampoo and soap. Mind you, you have to be careful when you clean jewellery.

I don't have the greatest track record, so this warning comes from the heart. One time I bent over the basin to clean my teeth while wearing sweetwater pearl earrings. They weren't madly expensive, but I liked them. When I looked up, one earring had disappeared down the

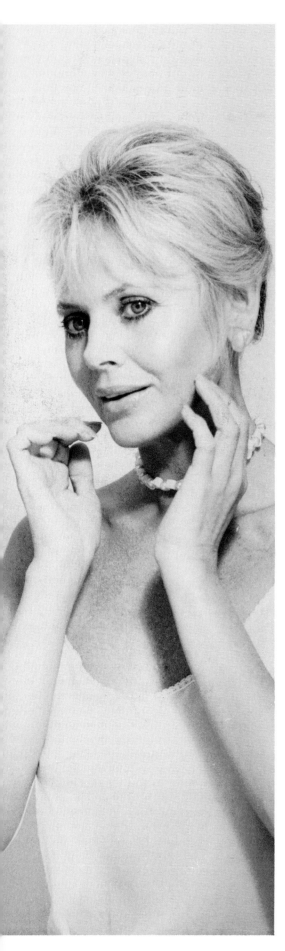

plughole. I lost a diamond stud earring down the shower, and one balmy night in Bangkok as I was sitting on a balcony talking I waved my hand, only to see a treasured ring go flying off into the depths of the murky River Klong.

So if you are anywhere near a sink or basin make sure the plug is in. If you are anywhere near a loo put the lid down. And if you are near a river keep your hands in your pockets.

Studs are safer, especially if they have a screw stem rather than push-on, but try to remember to take your diamonds out before you bath or shower. It's not necessarily the gushing water that dislodges them – it can happen when you wrap the towel around your head.

Gold chains and waterproof watches, whether gold or silver or other metal, respond well to good old soap and water. Use a mild soap, not perfumed toilet soap. I wouldn't use it on my body, so why use it on my jewels? Get a good lather going and rub the item between your hands. An old toothbrush is good for cleaning the fancy bits. Always brush the inside of rings where the claws are, because that's where dirt and soap tend to lodge.

You can clean ivory pieces in milk but don't let them soak. Never put semi-precious stones like jade, opals or pearls into jewel cleaner. They will disintegrate. Hard stones like amethysts and aquamarines are OK, though.

If in Doubt

1. Keep it simple, then you can't go wrong. Anyway, clear stones and simple, classic settings are always younger and prettier. Take a look at the Tiffany style.

2. Avoid jewellery that sticks out from your body and points and hangs on its own. It will get in the way during romantic encounters, get caught in coat sleeves and ruin your hair.

3. Educate the man in your life. Drop big hints and conjure up an extremely graphic image of the kind of stuff you like. That way, if he decides to splash out you won't be disappointed.

4. If you've got stubby, bitten nails, don't wear rings.

5. When you are tired of wearing your repertoire of jewellery, put it away, preferably in a safe. Pretend you don't have it for six months, then you will fall in love with it all over again.

6. Keep jewellery in separate bags. Don't bash it all together in a box. For instance, emeralds are very delicate stones and could easily be scratched by diamonds.

7. When you travel, never leave valuables behind in a hotel room because they won't be there when you get back. Don't try and hide them at the bottom of a suitcase, either – thieves know all the tricks and could teach you a few. It's better to carry everything in your handbag and keep it with you at all times.

Fake Is Fun

I'd never buy imitation classic diamonds or pearls, but in the summer I love to supplement my wardrobe with some cheap, festive, decorative pieces that are obvious fakes.

No one would mistake my pink 'pearls' for the real thing – they are very obviously plastic – but I love this necklace of pearls and pink ribbon strung together and the little matching shell-shape earrings. They add the finishing touch to my summer dresses.

If you want to go dramatic, try over-sized earrings like my black and red triangles. You can't wear much else with them because they're so dominant. Bangles and a necklace would definitely be too much, but they look great with a suit and hat, or even just a plain black dress.

They are heavy, though, which is why I definitely favour pierced ears. I only have one ear pierced, so I work with clip-on earrings and the pain at the end of the day can be excruciating. If you own stud earrings and want a change for summer, fake coral, fake jade, and fake pearls can look very pretty.

Small studs are the most flattering if you have a fat face, a double chin, or a scrawny neck. If you've got a heart-shaped face and short hair you can wear drop earrings down to your shoulders if you want to. If your hair is long and you want to wear drop earrings, put it up so it doesn't tangle with them.

If you need something elegant to wear with an evening dress, I'd suggest scouring antique shops for pretty diamanté and 1920s-style clips. They look expensive even though they're not, and can be very stylish.

If you're really intent on wearing a dramatic piece, say a gold chain with a single stone surrounded by diamonds, and you can't possibly afford the real thing, here are some pointers. Make sure your dress looks a million dollars. If it's a strikingly sophisticated gown that looks worthy of real jewels, then you'll be able to get away with it. Wear the same necklace with a wrinkled, cheap cloth suit and no one will believe it for a second.

Keep it simple. Just wear the necklace, perhaps with a matching pair of earrings, nothing more. Make sure the backs of the earrings aren't visible – they're a sure-fire way to spot a fake.

I'm not keen on body chains. To be honest, I had such a conservative upbringing that I always think chains around the ankle or waist look rather common. The only time I think they're fun is if you're on holiday and want to show off a tan and a super-trim body.

Better still, it can be romantic to pick a local bloom and stick it behind your ear. That's assuming you're holidaying in Hawaii or Barbados and not in Cornwall!

Although we rather flowered out in the 1960s, I'm quite partial to fabric fakes, especially nice silk ones. I'd stick a pretty flower in my hat band or in the breast pocket of a simple suit. Put a safety pin inside to hold it in place. A couple of blooms look good on a jacket lapel, too.

If last year's silk flowers look as though someone has sat on them, boil a pan of water and hold the flowers over it. Stay a good eight inches away from the water and gently shape the petals with your fingers over the steam. Let them dry naturally. You can revive any fabric flowers that way, and suede too.

Hair combs always look very tempting when they're jammed full of pearls and feathers and ribbons and beads, but in my experience they're not very practical. Combs in particular invariably slide out halfway through the evening when you are nowhere near a mirror. I use basic slides for convenience if I want to keep my hair back, but that's it.

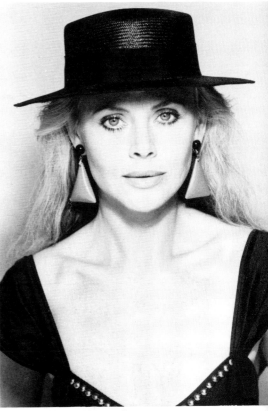

Fake jewellery is fun, and can give you and your wardrobe a new lease of life

15 / ATLANTIC CROSSINGS

Crossing the Atlantic or hopping down to Australia makes you learn a trick or two about travelling, especially when you know you have to face a barrage of photographers after a twelve-hour flight. I can't see the point of sitting in a chic suit, silk shirt and high heels when you will inevitably curl up in a ball and fall asleep. That's a sure way to arrive looking a wreck. If I plan to arrive wearing a silk shirt and suit, I stuff tissue paper up the shirt sleeves so it doesn't crease and carry the lot on to the plane in a hanging bag.

I always travel with a change of clothes, even on a car trip – either my favourite old khaki jumpsuit or an el cheapo jogging suit with zip-up top so I don't destroy my hair. As soon as they switch off that 'Fasten Seatbelt' sign on planes I nip into the loo, take everything off and change. Then I'm comfortable for the rest of the journey. Of course I always get the same comment 'Repairing the engine, are we?' to which I say, 'Yes we are, and we're going to make it safely, thank you very much.'

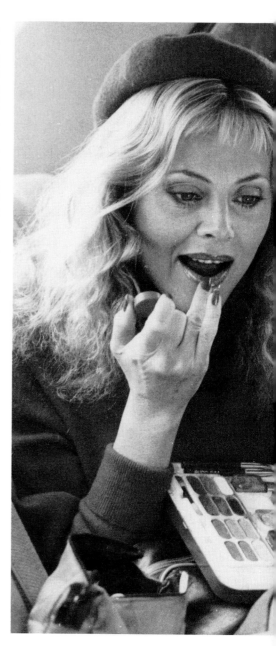

I always fly with my special Lone Ranger eye mask (see Chapter 3). Air stewardesses are always intrigued, so I can usually persuade them to fit it in the fridge during the flight. I cleanse every scrap of make-up off – everything but mascara – put lashings of moisturizer around my eyes, take a sleeping pill, pop in my earplugs and tell the stewardesses not to disturb me. The only thing I'm missing is that famous food, which I wouldn't touch anyway. Since flying dehydrates you, I bring a big bottle of mineral water which I swig throughout the journey, when I'm awake.

I aim for five hours' sleep on a twelve-hour flight, so that I don't feel wrecked the other end. Then when everyone is tucking into the crummy breakfast, I go in and hog the bathroom. I take my entire kit and wash my face, hands, underarms and any other place that needs freshening up, and come back totally refreshed with teeth brushed. Here's where the mask comes in – I retrieve it from the fridge and sit there with it on for ten minutes to cool my eyes down. You can wrap a newspaper round your face, but I just sit there oblivious to all the stares.

When I'm flying I really don't give a damn who is sitting next to me and I can put make-up on anywhere – in the back of a van, in a car, sitting in someone's lap, lying down. If I'm in a car I unfold the glove compartment and use it as a table while someone else drives (an old trick I learned when touring Sweden with a repertory company). When

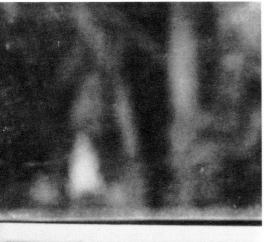

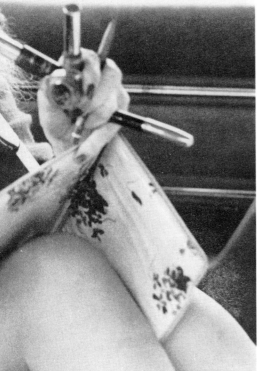

I'm flying I use the meal tray; cover it with paper towels from the bathroom, just as I would at home. A steady hand comes with practice.

Mini Travel Kit

I carry small sizes of everything I normally use at home. What I can't buy I decant into little bottles and jars saved from special offers. I never move without my Elizabeth Arden Eight Hour Cream – there are little pots of it scattered around my home – and I put it on my lips whenever I think of it.

Toothpaste and toothbrush are a must. I also carry eye shades, and because there are such things as babies on planes (poor unfortunate creatures) earplugs are the most important thing in the world. I recommend the pink, waxy kind rather than the white spongy ones. That little lot gives me the peace and tranquillity I need.

At the Other End

I put everything on hangers in the bathroom – the steam from the shower makes minor creases drop out. Of course a travel iron is a must. I pop a towel on the floor and give everything a once over before I wear it.

Boots take up lots of packing space. Make it work for you by stuffing them with anything soft – rolled up tights, bras, panties, even jeans or an evening bag.

Travelling Light

By nature I am the kind of person to whom travelling light means not carrying more than two suitcases. I've been known to go to Paris fully intending to buy clothes immediately, yet still lugging two suitcases jammed full of stuff that I don't wear. To be me and to survive with the bare minimum just isn't possible. But I can tell you what my bare minimum suitcase would contain should I ever be forced to resort to it:

1. A pair of jeans that can be glammed up for the evening. Black gabardine designer jeans or black leather are good because they can look exciting with a gold blouse, or a shimmery or leopard-print top.

With black high-heeled shoes they look, if not exactly elegant, certainly passable.

2. If I was going away for a fairly conservative weekend I would take a good tailor-made trouser suit. Trousers save wearing stockings. A black suit is smart but sexy and is good because you can take three or four different coloured shirts and they will also work with the jeans.

3. For short trips the real secret is to stick to one basic colour so that you don't need a multitude of accessories. If you have black shoes and a black handbag everything is interchangeable.

4. Also simple but definitely dramatic are a red shirt, red high-heeled shoes and red nylon socks (not stockings), which look very elegant and festive.

5. Alternatively I would take a short skirt and top. I like leopard-print in any shape and form. I think it's sexy and it's always been around, right through the thirties, forties and fifties, and to my mind it will never be passé. What's more, it looks equally good during the day or at night.

6. For comfort and relaxation a sweatsuit is a must. Sweatsuits are the most magnificent discovery – you can roll them up to pack them. I also love legwarmers.

7. If I am going somewhere cold I like to cosy up in a fur coat. It's not bulky to take because I put it in a hanging bag and carry it over my arm.

8. I don't need a nightie, and I take a pair of knickers for each day, plus one pair extra. I also travel everywhere with my silk teddy, my stockings and suspender belt. You never know!

9. I just take one handbag and never more jewellery than I can wear at once, otherwise I am bound to lose it. Hats are impossible to travel with so I just take the one I wear on my head.

10. Summer trips are easier – all you need for sensual dressing is a pair of shorts, a couple of T-shirts, a swimsuit, a bikini, a Victorian petticoat, and a lace overblouse, and you're all set.

The bathing suit can be worn like a leotard under the skirt at night with a big scarf round the middle. During the day you can wear the same outfit to the beach. Victorian petticoats are an absolute godsend, as are the little camisole tops that go with them. Tie a white chiffon scarf round your waist rather than a belt. If gold is your favourite metal, by all means wear gold accessories – shoes, handbag, chains.

Take a soft, straw hat that you can roll up and pack, not the brittle kind that falls apart. It might look good on a donkey with his ears sticking out but it's useless for the rest of us.

My Home Wardrobe System

I'm geared to packing at a moment's notice. I realize not everyone has a walk-in wardrobe but the principle still applies – it's easier to find things if you hang clothes graded by colour from white to black. I also grade by length within the colours from short to long – blouses, trousers, skirts, then evening gowns. I keep belts and sweaters packed in plastic bags and have separate drawers for stockings and tights, for matching bras and pants, for separate bras and pants, and for exercise gear (leotards, legwarmers, headbands), for handkerchiefs, and for gloves. I can find anything in seconds.

The Victorian petti look – I've always loved it

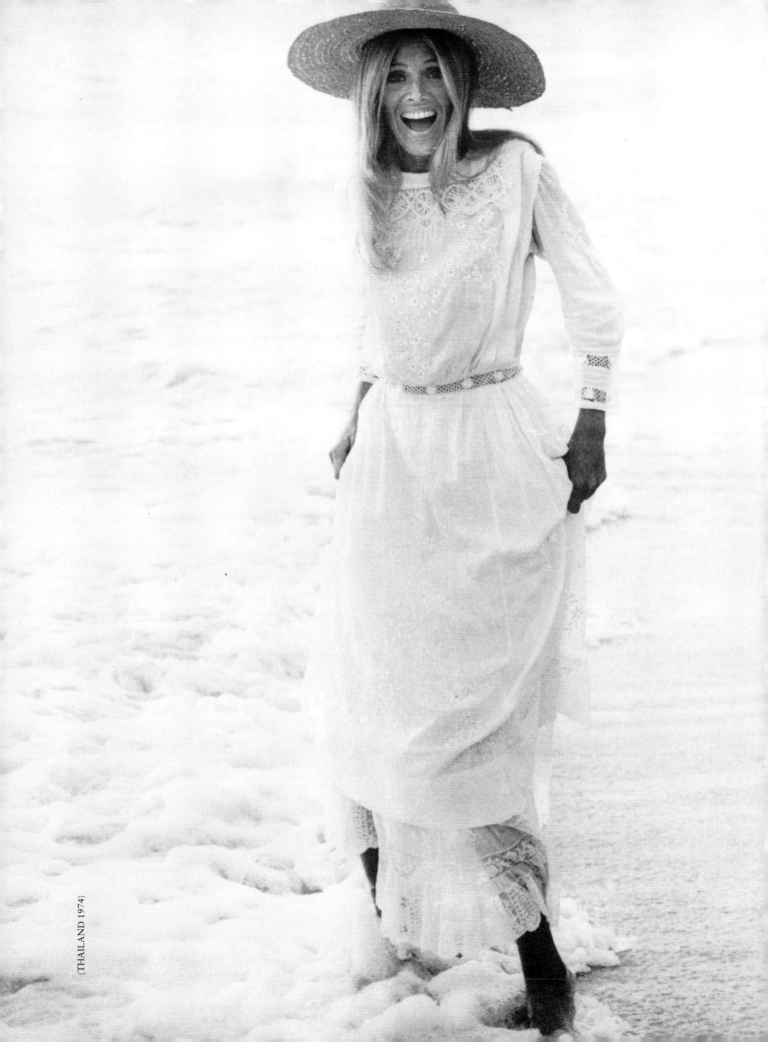

16/BEHIND THE BEDROOM DOOR

Men search for a mother/whore/wife/housekeeper/maid/mistress/lover all rolled into one. Whoever came up with that theory definitely had the right idea. I believe all men like to be seduced and that all men have slutty, tarty taste. Normally one should not generalize, but so far as sex is concerned I believe you can.

I have never made love to anyone older than I am today and I have no desire to. That's just the way I am. I don't think it is a sexual affliction – some people like red, some people like blue, I like men under forty. The oldest man I've ever made love to was my husband, Sellers, and I've never made love to anyone older since.

I matured very late. Not physically, but emotionally and mentally. It didn't happen gradually from the age of eighteen, it was literally 'bang' one day when I was in my thirties. Most of my sexual awareness and sensuality has surfaced since then.

Growing up in the 1950s guaranteed sexual hang-ups. There was so much emphasis on being a good girl, not 'putting out' as they say in America, keeping your legs together and oh, the horror and shame of all those shotgun weddings.

In some ways I was lucky in that I married an older man, and older men certainly help a young girl get over a lot of those emotional, intellectual, sexual, and sensual fears. But at the same time I think the older man creates some disturbance. The majority of young girls, myself included, are not physically ready really to enjoy sex. The physical apparatus is right but the mental attitude isn't. It doesn't matter who makes love to young girls, it could be Casanova himself, they are just not yet comfortable in their own bodies.

It can be very difficult for a vulnerable young girl to marry someone older and be thrown into a sexual relationship on a daily basis. Instead of her becoming more open and sensual, sex can turn into something she puts barriers up against and becomes almost afraid of. I think, in a way, that is what I did.

I had so many inhibitions that were so hard to get rid of. Some of them are still with me, I know, but I overcame most of them with a vengeance and I guess I went a little overboard at the same time which was, I think, understandable under the circumstances. Thanks to my hectic love life, I realize that I cannot claim to be an expert on long-term relationships. I haven't been married for ten years or even slept with the same man for ten years, but I do believe that I am sensitive and knowledgeable enough to project myself into that situation.

I know a lot of women in long-term relationships who started out

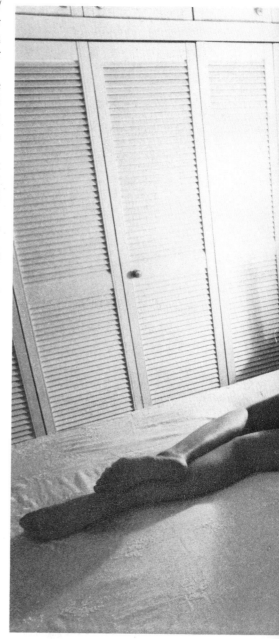

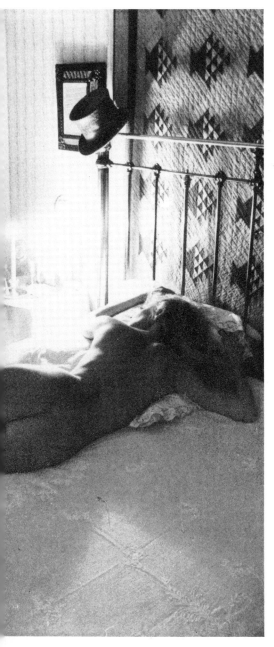

looking very sexy, wearing sensual clothes and painted fingernails, and then lost interest under the weight of the mundaneness of their day-to-day lives.

I do believe that despite the children, the breast-feeding, the dish-washing and chip fat smells, a woman can remain, or return to being, the sensual creature she was when she started. If things have gone flat in her relationship, she can't just sit and wonder why her man hasn't shown any interest in lovemaking for a month and comes up with weak excuses about being busy at the office. She's got to keep up her end if the relationship is going to stay alive.

But the problem doesn't always rest with the woman. It happened to me once. The man I lived with wouldn't make love to me, and like many women I immediately jumped to the conclusion that there was something wrong with me. It didn't occur to me that there might be something wrong with him. In reality the man in question had a major financial problem, and although he was in his early thirties and very active sexually, he simply lost his libido for a while. At times like that, rushing into your sexiest gear still won't turn him on and you will both end up feeling worse than ever. It's best just to give it a rest for a while.

I've learned a lot about sex and a lot about men in my travels, but I wouldn't want my whole life to be quite as 'adventurous' as it has been for the past few years. It's very tiring for one thing, but I also believe that when you find the right person it is wonderful to make a commitment. But commitment or no commitment, you should never stop working on the sensual side of your life.

I try hard not to shatter any illusions and tend to be very private about all the unglamorous beauty rituals I go through. It's nice, later on, to be able to reveal your naked self to the man you love and let him watch you strip away the layers of make-up. But for me that would be a very rare occurrence. I believe bathroom routines are private territory.

One famous film star obviously does not agree with me. I was at a party and asked for a guided tour of the house. The host escorted me to the master bedroom – a marvellous room with a huge, round bed in one corner, a big mirror, and an archway that I assumed led to a wardrobe. It didn't – it led to the bathroom complete with an absolutely gorgeous sunken bath and a toilet on a little throne. But there were no doors. No doors!

I was told that after fourteen years of marriage there are no secrets, but to me that isn't the point. It's not that I'm in favour of hiding in the

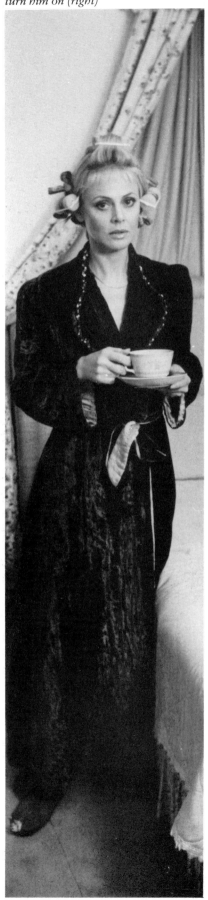

How to turn him off (below), and how to turn him on (right)

dark, though there are lots of adults who do. They undress in the bathroom and creep into bed with the light out and whatever might follow is always done in the pitch dark. Not me. I maintain that unless I can see the man I'm with, then he might as well be a gorilla. Besides, I think it's a total myth that women aren't visual creatures when it comes to sexual arousal. If you love someone, you want to look at them. Not just during sex, but if they are reading or watching TV. If you are at work all day it may be your only chance to see your lover.

I think you lose something if you make love with the lights out. You can share a lot through looks. A lot of feelings can come out, a lot of love.

Lighting to Make Love By

You couldn't read in my bedroom even if you wanted to. I have little Art Nouveau lamps and low, low lighting. For any woman not used to prancing around in the nude, it's a good way to hide a few imperfections.

If your man wants to read, let him have one of those horrible lamps that stick out on an arm, and make sure it's on a dimmer switch. Check that none of your lights cast awful sharp shadows and try soft pink light bulbs to give the room (and your skin) a bit of a rosy glow. The harshest form of lighting is fluorescent. I wouldn't have it anywhere, not even in the laundry room.

I have candles absolutely everywhere. I have them in my bathroom. I have them in my bedroom, I have them in my living room, summer and winter. People think it's permanently Christmas but candles are like flowers – whether your home is ultra-modern or rustic, they fit in perfectly. The kind I like best are those expensive smelly ones like Rigaud, but there are plenty of cheaper ones and you can put them into glasses or pretty containers.

Mood Makers

Before you commit yourself on the way you decorate your bedroom, decide what you want to happen in it.. Even if it's never happened before, design it around that fantasy and maybe it will happen! If you invite someone into a room where everything literally spells 'sex', that can be intimidating, but the mood of your bedroom can go a long way to enhance lovemaking.

My bedrooms in London and Los Angeles contrast dramatically. In London I picked pink and white Laura Ashley print bed linen. The whole look is very crisp and fresh and lends itself to light colour nightwear, more the schoolgirl-type, innocent look. In California my bedroom is altogether more dark and alluring, more thirties, and is perfect for anything from black stockings, suspender belts and high heels to Victorian lace nighties. Bear in mind the nightclothes you want to wear.

If your bedroom is large and you use it for more than sleeping, I'd move away from a strictly bedroom look. I have a cream satin quilted bedspread on my bed in Los Angeles. It has a big butterfly embroidered in the middle and matching pillows, and in daylight it doesn't look so instantly 'boudoir'. It's a large room and I feel quite comfortable working in it or sitting around chatting to my kids.

The one essential for everyone is a duvet. I don't care whether you live in London, Stockholm or Los Angeles, a duvet eliminates all that nasty bedmaking, not to mention the need for hot water bottles,

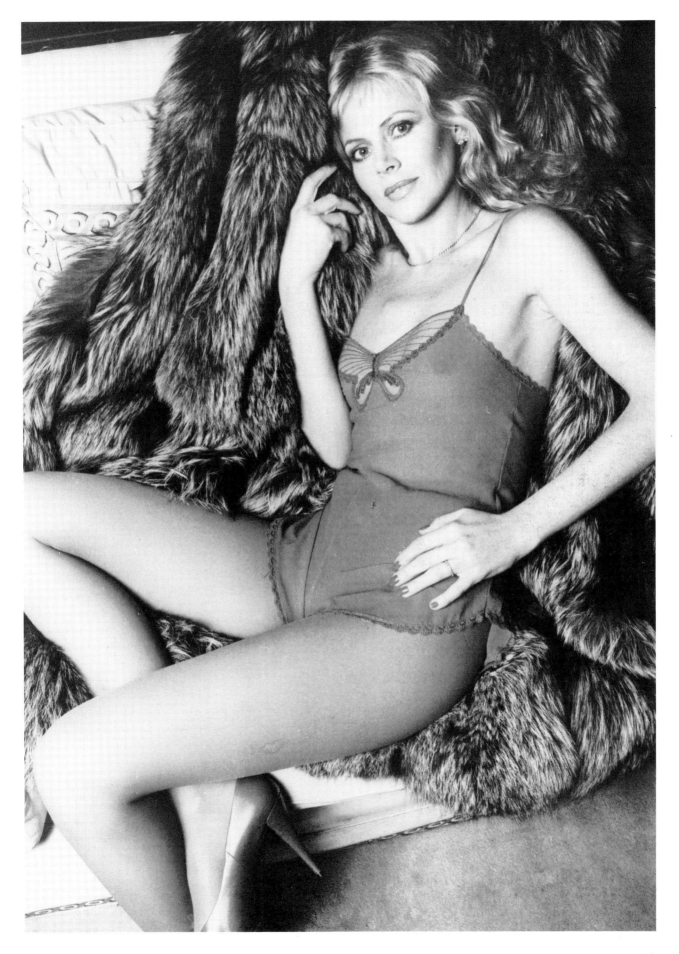

electric blankets and any of those other granny items I can't imagine using. If you have a duvet you will never be that cold. My family call them 'fluffies'. The feeling of a duvet next to your skin is infinitely more sensual than the feeling of a blanket, even one made of cashmere. Pure down is so phenomenally expensive that unless you are a multi-millionaire I'd buy a mixture of down and feathers or down and man-made fibre filling. Of course there is always an exception to every rule, and when it gets too warm for my fluffy a plain cotton sheet is all I use.

Make sure your mattress is on the firm side rather than soft, and never foam rubber, always interior sprung. Turn it at least twice a month, first sideways then lengthways, to keep it in good shape for lovemaking as well as sleeping.

To make your bedroom really inviting and feminine I'd always buy a frilly dust ruffle. It also means the man in your life won't have to look at your vacuum cleaner nozzle and your laundry bag, because they will be stashed under the bed and hidden from view. I'd also buy a fitted, white, quilted mattress cover, then top that with a fitted bottom sheet. Fitted sheets are a wonderful invention since you can never make a bed that neatly with the other kind, but for goodness sake measure carefully before you buy. If the sheet is too long it's OK, but if it's too short it's a disaster.

My Laura Ashley bed linens are reversible, so I can switch the emphasis from predominantly white with pink, to predominantly pink with white. They are pure cotton, which I love to feel against my skin. When they're new they tend to come out of the dryer looking like a rumpled suit, but after half a dozen washes the cotton softens up. I don't iron anything, because I don't have time. I just fluff them up and they look fine. Marks and Spencer bed linen is similar but cheaper. Alternatively, of course, you can buy a cotton/polyester mix and if you don't mind the feel of them they are more practical. They come out of the dryer looking as if they've just been ironed. I would never buy satin sheets, which look sexy but are too slippery.

Colour co-ordinated sheets and duvet cover are really all you need. Sometimes I will throw a very fine, see-through, Victorian lace spread over the whole lot for a more elegant touch. You don't *need* a bedspread with a duvet, but if you want to use one for effect just pop it on top.

Dressing Up to Undress

You can't go wrong with slut red nails and slut black lingerie, black stockings and black lace suspender belts. That goes for pleasing men of any age. You can be eighteen years old and kit yourself out in that stuff, but unless you're 100 per cent comfortable inside it will not come across as sensual but will probably look ridiculous. I believe one of the reasons younger men are attracted to older women is because older women are comfortable with that whole look and image, and that fulfils men's fantasies. When you get to forty you know yourself pretty well and you're at ease – hopefully – with pretty much anything.

It's no secret that in bed men are always very intrigued by the little girlie look, the schoolgirl-type with gymslip and white stockings. I could portray that look because physically and visually I can still look like a little girl, particularly in a dimly lit room, and it's a role I feel comfortable with.

I would personally never go to bed in a black rubber suit with cut-out nipples and a slit up my bum, because I wouldn't feel comfortable in it. I'm not ready for that yet. Maybe that's something to come, but to

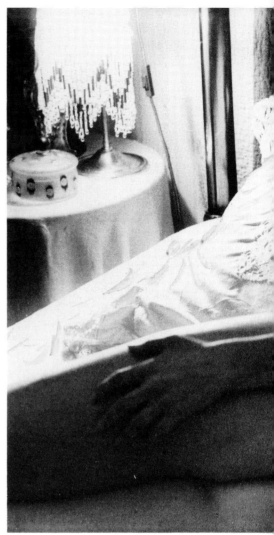

Above: Low lighting and pretty bed linens match a romantic mood

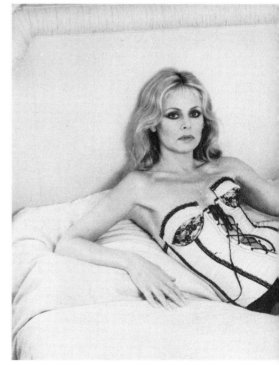

140

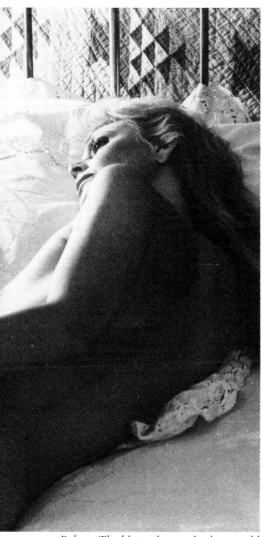

me that is not a sensual thing to go to bed in. Anything with cut-out bits is not sensual. To me it's dirty, and there's a difference between being sensual and sex-dirty. Not that sex-dirty is bad, but it's a different kind of feel and look from sensuality. I can't really see the average woman surprising her unsuspecting husband by suddenly stalking into the bedroom in stiletto heels and suspender belt and panties with a cut-out front. I just can't see it unless she gets drunk first. It would be too much of a shock for both of them.

Fifteen years ago the sexiest nightwear was baby dolls, but today the camisole or teddy has taken over and it's the perfect initiation into sexy gear. It's easy to put on, easy to take off, and has intriguing little press-studs underneath. Dramatic colours are the most effective. I own one black, one red and one white and I think you've got to go one way or the other, virginal or tarty. Black is obviously great on blondes, and black lacy bits are an instant turn-on.

Red is a good dramatic colour for blondes and brunettes alike. If your man is a raving sex maniac, go for black and red together – either red trimmed with black or black trimmed with red. Pink's good too (I have a pink waspie trimmed with black and that looks very sexy) but always avoid brash colours like turquoise and orange and sharp blue – they're not sensual and are actually off-putting.

At the other end of the image scale there are wonderful second-hand Victorian nightdresses which mean you can creep into bed looking like a child out of a story book. Sometimes that makes you feel better, but I'm not so sure it makes him feel better. It's a pretty way to go to bed, though.

I've only been with one man who wore pyjamas – silk pyjamas in fact. But there is nothing about pyjamas that turns me on and that goes for the old idea of women wearing the jackets – that's strictly for the movies. I'm so tired of that look and I don't even think it's a turn-on.

Dressing-gowns can be very sexy, but Japanese kimonos are often a cheap, flattering alternative. Pure silks, cottons, and satins are very sensual. Even a cheap thin Chinese silk looks good; it's very contour-revealing – you might as well be naked, but you're not.

I'd avoid candlewick unless it's for warmth. It's better suited to bedspreads. I'd also avoid kimonos in that stiff, thick, artificial satin, which isn't soft enough to be sensual. I'm not keen on nylon although there are pretty things made in it, so I'd just avoid the sharp, obnoxious colours like shocking pink, bright baby blues, and acid yellows. They don't flatter anyone.

I love towelling, but not the thin, threadbare, scratchy kind. It has to be lush, soft, and very thick. The Ritz Hotel in Paris supplies guests with apricot terry robes and those are very sensual. I'd have two robes – a warm, practical, fluffy towelling one and something more glamorous. The prettiest colours are white, black, champagne, or skin. If you are older, light peach does wonders and makes you look about seventeen. Red, once again, is a very enticing colour but if you're older or on the large side, I'd stay with black or beige.

A Few Tips

1. Full-length kimonos work well if you are short, fairly squat, and have bulging thighs, but your good features are a nice cleavage and slim ankles. You can arrange kimonos so they fall open sexily at the front yet cover the rest.

2. Short kimonos are ideal if you've got a good figure, not thin necessarily, but well-proportioned. If you've got good breasts – they

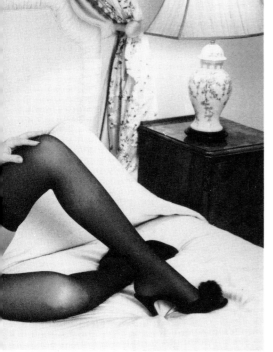

Below: The blatantly sexy look – would you dare to try it?

* If you don't have your period but are worried about what we can politely call leakage during exercise class or in the bedroom, use a slim tampon. If you're in the bedroom, make sure the string doesn't show and keep it in until you get into bed, then pull it out in the dark. One has to be practical.

* The basic essential to sensual lovemaking is that you be impeccably clean. It's a turnoff to spend the day running around sweating and then leap straight into bed. Clean, fresh body sweat is fine though.

don't have to be large – you can afford to show them off. Wear little panties and nothing else underneath, then every time you bend over you will show lots of leg and cleavage.

3. Wear an Empire-style nightie as a dressing-gown if you have lots to hide and only one thing to show – your breasts. It will be tight under the bust so you won't need a bra.

4. If the tops of your arms bulge a bit, wear something sheer like cotton voile which looks transparent but covers what you don't want to be seen. You can also buy a long-sleeved style and cut and hem the sleeves to just above the elbow.

5. If you like the little girl look, shorten a Victorian nightgown and wear it around the house as a dressing-gown.

Getting Down to the Bare Essentials

I wouldn't make it into a studied ritual – to look good taking your clothes off you have to do it the way it feels natural. Even if you know he's watching, I'd stand sideways and move as elegantly and prettily as possible. If you've got a zipper it's nice and alluring to ask your man to unzip you.

Read his mood. If he's thrown his clothes off and jumped into bed you know he's going to want something fast, in which case maybe you should simply follow his lead and forget everything else. It's a common complaint from men that they loathe women disappearing into the bathroom for two hours. They mind even more at night than they do in the morning, and it's not just a matter of waiting for sex, they just want you there with them.

If you are wearing stockings and a suspender belt show them off by all means, but tights aren't that pretty or sexy. Either keep your robe handy so you can slip into it fast, or, better still, retire to the bathroom to freshen up.

Brush your hair, brush your teeth, wipe off a little make-up if you feel you are wearing too much. Wash your private parts, spritz talc under your arms and around the tops of your thighs. Keep a pair of high-heeled slippers in your bathroom or pop your shoes back on with your robe. If I come home alone my shoes are always the first thing to come off, but with a man around they are the last thing to go. Men love to see women in high heels.

Dressing up for bed is fun, but never forget that the nicest and ultimately most sensual feeling of all is the feeling of your skin and his skin. At the end of the day – providing you have done your beauty homework – nothing stirs like a bit of flesh!

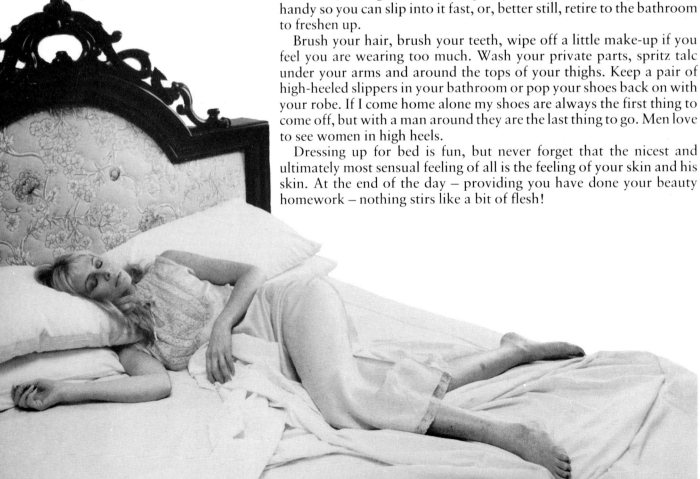

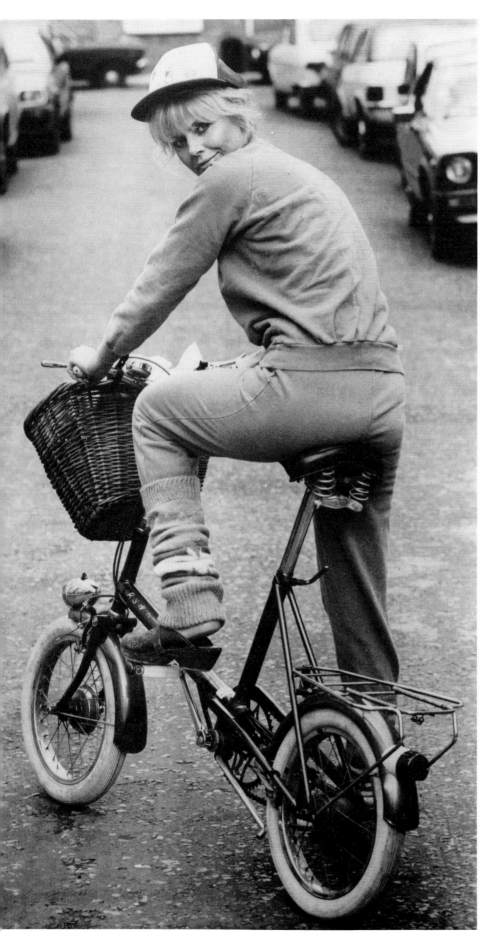

INDEX